MICROBIOLOGY

for the

Boards and Wards

Other books in the Boards and Wards series:

Notice: The indications and dosages of all drugs in this book have been recommended in the medical literature and conform to the practices of the general community. The medications described do not necessarily have specific approval by the Food and Drug Administration for use in the diseases and dosages for which they are recommended. The package insert for each drug should be consulted for use and dosage as approved by the FDA. Because standards for usage change, it is advisable to keep abreast of revised recommendations, particularly those concerning new drugs.

MICROBIOLOGY
for the
Boards and Wards

Carlos Ayala, MD
Clinical Fellow in Otology and Laryngology
Harvard Medical School
Resident in Otolaryngology
Harvard Otolaryngology Residency Program
Boston, Massachussetts

Brad Spellberg, MD
Resident in Internal Medicine
Harbor-UCLA Medical Center
Torrance, California

b

**Blackwell
Science**

©2001 by Carlos Ayala and Brad Spellberg

Editorial Offices:
Commerce Place, 350 Main Street, Malden, Massachusetts 02148, USA
Osney Mead, Oxford OX2 0EL, England
25 John Street, London WC1N 2BL, England
23 Ainslie Place, Edinburgh EH3 6AJ, Scotland
54 University Street, Carlton, Victoria 3053, Australia

Other Editorial Offices:
Blackwell Wissenschafts-Verlag GmbH, Kurfürstendamm 57, 10707 Berlin, Germany
Blackwell Science KK, MG Kodenmacho Building, 7-10 Kodenmacho Nihonbashi, Chuo-ku, Tokyo 104, Japan
Iowa State University Press, A Blackwell Science Company, 2121 S. State Avenue, Ames, Iowa 50014-8300, USA

Distributors:

USA
Blackwell Science, Inc.
Commerce Place
350 Main Street
Malden, Massachusetts 02148
(Telephone orders: 800-215-1000 or
781-388-8250; fax orders: 781-388-8270)

Canada
Login Brothers Book Company
324 Saulteaux Crescent
Winnipeg, Manitoba R3J 3T2
(Telephone orders: 204-837-2987)

Australia
Blackwell Science Pty, Ltd.
54 University Street
Carlton, Victoria 3053
(Telephone orders: 03-9347-0300;
fax orders: 03-9349-3016)

Outside North America and Australia
Blackwell Science, Ltd.
c/o Marston Book Services, Ltd.
P.O. Box 269
Abingdon
Oxon OX14 4YN
England
(Telephone orders: 44-01235-465500;
fax orders: 44-01235-465555)

Acquisitions: Beverly Copland
Development: Julia Casson
Production: Irene Herlihy
Manufacturing: Lisa Flanagan

Marketing Manager: Toni Fournier
Typeset by Software Services
Printed and bound by Capital City Press

Printed in the United States of America
01 02 03 04 5 4 3 2 1

The Blackwell Science logo is a trade mark of Blackwell Science Ltd., registered at the United Kingdom Trade Marks Registry

Library of Congress Cataloging-in-Publication Data
Ayala, Carlos, MD.
    Microbiology for the boards and wards/by Carlos Ayala and Brad Spellberg.
        p.; cm.
    Includes bibliographical references and index.
    ISBN 0-632-04576-0
    1. Medical microbiology—Examinations, questions, etc. I. Spellberg, Brad. II. Title.
    [DNLM: 1. Microbiology—Examination Questions. 2. Antibiotics—therapeutic
    use—Examination Questions. 3. Communicable Diseases—Examination Questions.
    QW 18.2 A973m 2001]
    QR46 .A96 2001
    616'.01'076—dc21
                                                                    2001025022

TABLE OF CONTENTS

TABLES

ABBREVIATIONS

↑/↓	increases or high/decreases or low
→	causes/leads to/analysis shows
CXR	chest x-ray
CNS	central nervous system
Dx	diagnosis
dz	disease
1°/2°	primary/secondary
GNC	gram negative cocci
GNR	gram negative rods
GPC	gram positive cocci
GPR	gram positive rods
hrs	hours
infxn	infection
lmtd	limited
pt(s)	patient(s)
Tx	treatment
μl	microliter
yrs	years (old)

PREFACE

In this book, descriptions of microorganisms are broken into eight categories: appearance, lab assays, virulence factors, epidemiology, clinical diseases, treatment, resistance, and prophylaxis. We do not intend a complete microbiological description of each pathogen. Instead, we provide information in each category only as it relates to testable USMLE material. Thus, you will frequently see "none" or "none significant" listed under the virulence factor section. This doesn't literally mean that there are no virulence factors associated with the organism. Instead it means there are no virulence factors you will be asked about on the boards exam. At the end of each section of organisms (e.g., gram positive cocci), we include summary tables listing the key characteristics of each organism for ease of rapid review.

The description of antibiotics is similarly broken into five sections, including mechanism, resistance, toxicities, cidal/static, and spectrum of coverage. Again, we focus only on information that is important for the USMLE exams.

ACKNOWLEDGMENTS

The authors would like to offer their most sincere thanks to Dr. Samuel French, Professor of Pathology at the UCLA School of Medicine and the Harbor–UCLA Department of Pathology. Dr. French provided all of the microbiology images for this book. He is a paragon of academic excellence, a true gentleman and scholar, who has throughout his career selflessly taught innumerable residents and students.

I. BASIC CONCEPTS

A. Bacteria

1. **Bacteria are prokaryotes**: single-cell organisms having no internal organelles

2. Almost all bacteria have cell walls, which are thick structures composed of a cross-linked glycopeptide called **peptidoglycan**, providing support for the cell

3. Bacteria also have an outer lipid envelope surrounding the cell wall, **composed of a glycolipid conjugate called lipopolysaccharide (LPS)**

4. **Gram stain**

   a. The gram stain is a 2-step process capable of staining different bacteria either purple or red depending upon the type of cell wall and lipid envelope surrounding the cell

   b. In step 1, a purple dye is added to the bacteria which is avidly adherent to the peptidoglycan of the cell wall, and then alcohol is added to wash away non-adherent purple dye

   c. In step 2, a red stain is added to the bacteria

   d. Gram positive organisms have thick peptidoglycan walls that avidly bind the purple dye, and which do not release the dye when alcohol is added

   e. Gram negative organisms have thin peptidoglycan walls that are rinsed clean of the purple dye by the alcohol, allowing the cells to be colored by the red counter-stain

   f. **Thus gram positive organisms stain purple, while gram negative organisms stain red**

5. Some bacteria have outer polysaccharide capsules surrounding the LPS envelope, which typically serve to protect the bacteria from host immune cells

6. **Atypical bacteria are those that cannot be identified by gram staining**

7. **Many atypical bacteria are "intracellular pathogens,"** meaning they live inside human cells, which enables them to cause disease

8. Intracellular pathogens have altered cell wall and envelope structures, some have unique lipids called mycolic acids (*Mycobacteria*), and some have no cell walls at all (*Mycoplasma*)

9. **Another kind of atypical bacteria are the spirochetes,** long, spiral-shaped bacteria which move with a corkscrew motion and tend to be extracellular pathogens

10. Flagella are long processes composed of microtubules that extend from the end of a bacteria, which are powered by ATP and are capable of making rapid, whip-like motions to propel the bacteria forward

11. Fimbriae are long glycoprotein extensions from the cell membrane that serve as adhesins to host surfaces, allowing bacterial colonization of a host

12. Infection versus colonization

   a) **Colonization is the peaceful coexistence of bacteria with a mammalian host,** for example *Staphylococcus aureus* living as a commensal organism on our skin

   b) Infection represents an invasive, damaging process initiated by the bacteria, for example cellulitis

   c) It can be very difficult in some clinical situations to determine whether a bacteria is only colonizing a host, and therefore does not need to be treated with antibiotics, or whether it is causing actual disease

   d) **The most reliable marker for infection versus colonization is the host inflammatory response,** that is, bacteria are present in both situations, but host inflammation is only present in infection, not in colonization

B. Fungi

1. **Fungi are eukaryotes,** meaning they have a nucleus and internal organelles separated from the cytoplasm by internal membranes

2. **Fungi all have cell walls,** often composed of complex glycoproteins such as chitin and mannoprotein

3. The chemical composition of fungal cell membranes is distinct from animal cell membranes: **while animal cell membranes contain cholesterol, fungal cell membranes contain ergosterol**

4. Some fungi grow as yeast, which are unicellular spherical forms that reproduce by budding

5. Other fungi grow as molds, which are conglomerates of multicellular, long, filamentous forms called hyphae

6. Still other fungi are called dimorphic because they can grow as yeast or molds depending upon the environment

7. Like a gram stain for bacteria, **the most useful laboratory stain for detecting fungi is the silver stain**—on a silver stain the background tissue appears light blue-green, while the fungi stain dark black

C. Protozoa

1. **Protozoa are unicellular eukaryotes** of the kingdom Protista

2. **Medically important protozoa are all parasites, meaning they live in humans and cause disease** (as opposed to commensal organisms which live on or in humans but do not cause disease)

3. Protozoa do not have cell walls

4. Many protozoa have complex life cycles involving phase changes in their cellular structure

5. Trophozoites are the forms of protozoa which are motile, whereas cysts are their tough stationary-phase form which allow them to survive in harsh external environments

D. Helminths

1. **Helminths are worms** of the kingdom Animalia

2. Helminths are thus **multicellular animals**, and the medically important ones are also parasites

3. Helminths can be divided into flatworms (platyhelminths, platy- = flat) and roundworms (nematodes)

4. Flatworms can be further divided into flukes (also called trematodes) and tapeworms (cestodes)

5. The stool ova and parasite (O&P) test is the classic way to identify worms in an infected patient

E. Viruses

1. Viruses are non-living automatons that hijack living cells and force cellular machinery to replicate the virus

2. Viruses contain a genome composed of RNA or DNA, a variety of structural proteins that form the viral core and viral capsid, and some contain lipid envelopes

3. Viral RNA can either be double-stranded or single-stranded in the viral genome, and single-stranded RNA can either be positive strand or negative strand

    a. Positive strand viral RNA directly codes for viral proteins (equivalent to mRNA)

    b. Negative strand viral RNA must be replicated to the complementary positive strand before transcription is possible

    c. Thus viruses whose genomes consist of negative strand RNA must carry within the viral capsid an RNA polymerase to convert the negative strand to a positive strand if viral replication is to occur

    d. Retroviruses have RNA genomes but convert the RNA into DNA prior to viral replication

    e. Thus, like negative-strand RNA viruses, retroviruses also carry a special viral polymerase, called reverse transcriptase, within their capsid

4. Viral susceptibility to sterilizing agents such as alcohol and halogenated chemicals depends on the presence or absence of the viral envelope

5. Non-enveloped viruses (called naked viruses) are highly resistant to chemical destruction, while enveloped viruses are more susceptible

II. BACTERIA

A. Gram Positive Cocci (GPC)

1. *Staphylococcus*

    a. *S. aureus*

        1) Appearance: **GPC in clusters** ("Staphylo-" means "grape-like" in Greek, refers to classic grape-cluster appearance), **colonies have golden hue**

        2) Lab assays: **coagulase positive** (secretes coagulase enzyme → clots serum), catalase positive (secretes catalase enzyme → H_2O_2 → $H_2O + O_2$), β-hemolytic (see Section 2. *Streptococci*)

        3) Virulence factors:

            a) Protein A is a cell-wall protein that binds to the constant region of IgG antibodies, preventing their variable regions from binding antigen

b) Enterotoxin

    i) Pre-formed exotoxin secreted in the intestines (entero = gut), heat resistant

    ii) Causes food-poisoning gastroenteritis, typified by nausea, vomiting, diarrhea, **within 8 hr of food consumption**

    iii) One variant is the Toxic Shock Syndrome Toxin (TSST)

        a)) A superantigen, binds to a constant region of the T cell receptor, non-specifically activating T lymphocytes resulting in unregulated inflammation

        b)) Acquired from contaminated tampons in menstruating women or from infected wounds

        c)) Leads to systemic hypotension, tachycardia

c) Exfoliatin

    i) Also a superantigen, causes "*Staphylococcus Scalded Skin Syndrome*" (SSSS), widespread superficial epidermal exfoliation seen almost exclusively in children

    ii) **Of little clinical consequence**, exfoliation is too superficial to be dangerous, and SSSS resolves quickly with antibiotics

4) Epidemiology: human skin flora, colonizes the nares, intertriginous areas, and areas of diseased skin such as psoriatic patches, transmission by direct contact and fomites

5) Clinical Diseases:

a) Skin infections: include cellulitis, folliculitis, local skin abscess (i.e. furuncle/carbuncle)

b) Bacteremia: **commonly due to intravenous drug abuse (IVDA), post-surgical, via wounds, or nosocomial via intravenous catheters**

c) Endocarditis: causes **acute, severe disease NOT subacute indolent disease**

d) Osteomyelitis

e) Pneumonia: **classically seen during the resolution phase of a prior viral pneumonia,** the patient is getting better and then all of a sudden relapses with sever cough and fevers, **multilobar pneumonia can also be seen in endocarditis due to septic emboli**

6) Treatment: 1st generation cephalosporin, β-lactamase resistant penicillin (e.g., methicillin), or vancomycin for Methicillin Resistant *S. aureus* (MRSA)

7) Resistance:

   a) β-lactamase: a ubiquitous plasma-encoded enzyme that inactivates the β-lactam ring common to all penicillins, treatment requires use of 1st generation cephalosporin, a β-lactamase resistant penicillin (e.g., methicillin), or addition of a β-lactamase inhibitor (e.g., clavulonic acid)

   b) Penicillin Binding Protein (PBP): a mutation in the usual protein bound by penicillins makes *S. aureus* resistant to even methicillin (MRSA), requiring the use of vancomycin

8) Prophylaxis: strict contact isolation and hand-washing

b. *S. epidermidis*

1) Appearance: GPC in clusters, colonies appear white on petri dish

2) Lab assays: **coagulase negative, novobiocin sensitive** (killed by novobiocin), catalase positive

3) Virulence factors: mucopolysaccharide (slime) allowing adhesion to plastic surfaces

4) Epidemiology: ubiquitous human skin flora

5) Clinical Diseases:

   a) Bacteremia: **nosocomial infections via intravenous catheters**

   b) Endocarditis: risk greatest for prosthetic valves within 6 months of valve replacement

   c) Prosthesis: bacteremia secondary to line infections can seed any plastic prosthetic

6) Treatment: vancomycin frequently required

7) Resistance: intrinsically resistant to most antibiotics

8) Prophylaxis: sterility during surgery and line placement

c. *S. saprophyticus*

1) Appearance: GPC in clusters, colonies appear white on petri dish

TABLE 1	Summary of *Staphylococcus spp.*			
	APPEARANCE	**LAB**	**VIRULENCE**	**EPIDEM.**
aureus	GPC clusters; **Gold** colonies	**Coagulase** ⊕	Toxins	Colonizes skin
epidermidis	GPC clusters; White colonies	Coagulase –; Novobiocin sensitive	**Plastic** adhesins	Colonizes skin
saprophyticus	GPC clusters; White colonies	Coagulase –; **Novobiocin resistant**	Mucosal adhesins	Colonizes GU mucosa

2) Lab assays: **coagulase negative, novobiocin resistant,** catalase positive

3) Virulence factors: epithelial adhesins

4) Epidemiology: genitourinary mucosa flora

5) Clinical Diseases: UTI

6) Treatment: Bactrim or fluoroquinolones

7) Resistance: intrinsically resistant to most penicillins

8) Prophylaxis: none

2. *Streptococcus*

α-hemolytic *Streptococci*

* α = partial hemolysis
* Forms green zone around colonies on blood agar petri dish due to partial degradation of red blood cells

  a. *S. pneumonia*

  1) Appearance: **GPC in pairs** (also known as diplococci)

  2) Lab assays: **susceptible to bile, deoxycholate, and optochin, quellung reaction positive** (swelling of polysaccharide capsule in presence of immune serum), catalase negative (**all *Streptococci* are catalase negative**)

  3) Virulence factors:

  a) IgA protease: degrades IgA in mucosal secretions

  b) Polysaccharide capsule: inhibits phagocytosis

4) Epidemiology:

a) Colonizes oropharynx in up to 50% of people

b) Host factors are crucial to allowing infection: **splenectomy, HIV, malnutrition, alcoholism, chronic lung disease, nephrotic syndrome, multiple myeloma, or in general, anything that inhibits host antibody responses markedly increases host susceptibility to *S. pneumonia***

5) Clinical Diseases:

a) Pneumonia (**#1 cause of community acquired pneumonia**), often with bacteremia

b) Meningitis (**#1 cause**)

c) Otitis media/Sinusitis

d) Bronchitis

6) Treatment: Penicillins, cephalosporins, macrolides, extended spectrum quinolones (e.g., levofloxacin)

7) Resistance:

a) Increasing resistance to penicillins due to altered Penicillin Binding Protein

b) High level resistance to 3rd generation cephalosporins is rare but increasing

8) Prophylaxis:

a) Pneumovax® is a polyvalent polysaccharide vaccine composed of capsular antigens from 23 *S. pneumo* isotypes

b) **Pneumovax should be given to all people ≥65 years old, all patients without spleens, and all patients with chronic debilitating illnesses** (e.g., heart failure, lung diseases, cirrhosis, renal failure, cancers, alcoholism, etc.)

b. Viridans group *Streptococci* (Viridans derives from the Latin word for "green," named for their α-hemolysis, refers to a number of different relatively avirulent *Strep* species)

1) Appearance: GPC in chains

2) Lab assays: **resistant to bile, deoxycholate, and optochin, quellung reaction negative**, catalase negative

3) Virulence factors: none significant

4) Epidemiology: human mouth flora

5) Clinical Diseases: endocarditis, **keys to diagnosis are history of poor dentition or recent dental procedures**

6) Treatment: penicillin + aminoglycoside, or 3rd gen. cephalosporin

7) Resistance: unusual

8) Prophylaxis: ampicillin prior to dental procedures, good dentition

β-hemolytic *Streptococci*

- β = complete hemolysis, forms clear zone around colonies on blood agar petri dish

- **Lancefield system: a subclassification of β-hemolytic *Streptococci* based upon the C-carbohydrate in the organism's cell wall**—only β-hemolytic *Strep* are classified by this system, so the terms Group A, Group B, or Group D *Strep* always refer to β-hemolytic *Strep*

- Groups C, E–G are rarely pathogenic and are not discussed

a. *S. pyogenes* (Group A Strep)

1) Appearance: GPC in chains

2) Lab assays: **bacitracin sensitive**, catalase negative

3) Virulence factors:

a) **M protein**: an anti-phagocytic component of the polysaccharide capsule, polymorphisms in the M protein allow subclassification of Group A *Strep* to identify individual strains—antibody to one form of M-protein provides immunity only to that particular strain of Group A Strep

b) Streptolysin O causes β-hemolysis, immune response to it generates an antibody commonly assayed for, to detect the presence of Group A Strep, called the **anti-streptolysin O (ASO) antibody**

c) Exotoxin A & B: A is a superantigen, while B causes the tissue necrosis seen in necrotizing fasciitis

d) **Erythrogenic toxin causes scarlet fever**

4) Epidemiology: frequently colonizes human skin, occasionally the oropharynx

5) Clinical Diseases:

a) Pharyngitis—classic Strep throat, can progress to otitis/sinusitis

b) Cellulitis/impetigo/erysipelas

c) Necrotizing fasciitis: **the classic flesh-eating virus, which, ironically, is not a virus and does not "eat" the flesh** (it necrotizes tissue by secreting exotoxin B)

d) Post-streptococcal glomerulonephritis: **immune complex deposition** causes rapidly progressive nephritic syndrome, although acute renal failure develops, it is typically self-limiting—note, this occurs 2–3 weeks after the resolution of any Strep infection (cellulitis, pharyngitis, or other)

e) Rheumatic fever: due to an **immunologic cross-reaction (molecular mimicry)** with a Group A Strep antigen, resulting in heart valve damage, fever, rash, migratory polyarthritis, choreiform movements, with elevated ASO titers—the disease occurs 2 weeks after a Group A Strep infection, and can be prevented by antibiotic treatment within the first week of infection

f) Scarlet fever: a self-limiting exfoliative disorder due to erythrogenic toxin, resulting in the classic sandpaper-like maculopapular eruption

6) Treatment: 100% of strains susceptible to penicillin

7) Resistance: none

8) Prophylaxis: antibiotic therapy prevents glomerulonephritis and rheumatic fever

b. *S. agalactiae* (Group B Strep)

1) Appearance: GPC in chains, occasionally in pairs

2) Lab assays: **bacitracin resistant, hydrolyzes hippurate, CAMP factor positive** (causes synergistic hemolysis with *Staph. aureus*, a rapid CAMP factor assay is available), catalase negative

3) Virulence factors: an antiphagocytic capsule

4) Epidemiology:

a) Colonizes female genitourinary tract

b) **Group B Strep in the urine is a marker for high organism burden**

c) **Prolonged rupture of membranes is the key risk factor to neonatal transmission**

d) **Premature infants are at increased risk for infection**

5) Clinical Diseases: neonatal bacteremia and meningitis (it is the most common cause in neonates)

6) Treatment: penicillins +/– aminoglycoside

7) Resistance: none

8) Prophylaxis: treat pregnant women colonized with Group B Strep with ampicillin during labor, and treat women with prolonged rupture of membranes

c. *S. bovis* (Group D Strep)

1) Appearance: GPC in chains

2) Lab assays: **resistant to bile, hydrolyze esculin** (produce black pigment on bile/esculin agar), **susceptible to hypertonic saline** (note: this differentiates them from *Enterococcus*, which used to be classified as Group D Strep, see below), catalase negative

3) Virulence factors: none significant

4) Epidemiology: human intestinal flora

5) Clinical Diseases: bacteremia and endocarditis—note, up to 50% of patients with *S. bovis* endocarditis have an underlying colon cancer that allowed the organism to translocate into the bloodstream, **so always think colon cancer if this organism comes up on the boards**

6) Treatment: penicillins

7) Resistance: none

8) Prophylaxis: none

γ-hemolytic *Streptococci*

- γ = lack of hemolysis

- Strains from a number of species can be γ-hemolytic, including Viridans Strep (usually α-hemolytic), *Strep. bovis* (usually β-hemolytic), as well as *Enterococcus* (see below)

3. *Enterococci*

a. *E. faecalis* & *E. faecium*

1) Appearance: GPC in chains & pairs

2) Lab assays: **resistant to bile, hydrolyze esculin** (produce black pigment on bile/esculin agar), **resistant to hypertonic saline**

3) Virulence factors: none significant

TABLE 2	Summary of *Streptococcus & Enterococcus spp.*			
	APPEARANCE	**LAB**	**VIRULENCE**	**EPIDEM.**
Streptococcus spp.				
pneumonia	GPC **pairs**	α-hemolytic **quellung positive**	Capsule	**Splenectomy**, HIV+, alcohol, chronic disease
viridans	GPC chains	α-hemolytic **resistant to bile/optochin/ deoxycholate**	None	**Dental procedures cause infxn**
pyogenes	GPC chains	β-hemolytic **bacitracin sensitive**	**M Protein, streptolysin O**	Skin flora
agalactiae	GPC chains	β-hemolytic, **bacitracin resistant, CAMP factor positive**	Capsule	**Female GU** tract, **neonatal infections**
bovis	GPC chains	β or γ-hemolytic, **resistant to bile, hydrolyzes esculin, inhibited by hypertonic saline**	None	Lives in colon, **colon cancer** predisposes to infection
Enterococcus spp.				
faecalis/ faecium	GPC chains/pairs	α, β, or γ-hemolytic, **resistant to bile, hydrolyzes esculin, resistant to hypertonic saline**	None	Intestinal flora, participates in **polymicrobial infections**

4) Epidemiology: human intestinal flora

5) Clinical Diseases:

    a) UTI

    b) Biliary infections (e.g., cholangitis)

    c) Abdominal/pelvic abscesses

    d) Endocarditis

TABLE 3	Laboratory Summary of Gram Positive Cocci			
	APPEARANCE	**CATALASE**	**HEMOLYSIS**	**UNIQUE PROPERTY**
Staphylococcus spp.				
Aureus	Clusters	⊕	β	Coagulase ⊕, gold colonies
Epidermidis	Clusters	⊕	γ	Novobiocin sensitive
Saprophyticus	Clusters	⊕	γ	Novobiocin resistant
Streptococcus spp.				
Pneumonia	Pairs	–	α	Quellung reaction ⊕
Viridans	Chains	–	α, γ	Resist bile/ deoxycholate/ optochin
Pyogenes	Chains	–	β	Bacitracin sensitive
Agalactiae	Chains	–	β	Bacitracin resistant, CAMP ⊕
Bovis	Chains	–	β or γ	Resist bile, lysed by hypertonic saline
Enterococcus spp.				
Faecalis/ faecium	Chains/pairs	–	α, β, or γ	Resist bile & hypertonic saline

6) Treatment:

   a) *E. faecalis*: ampicillin, extended-spectrum penicillins (e.g., piperacillin), imipenem, or vancomycin, with aminoglycoside for synergy

   b) *E. faecium*: vancomycin with aminoglycoside for synergy, **beware of Vancomycin-Resistant *Enterococcus* (VRE), which can only be treated with linezolid or quinupristin/dalfopristin (Synercid®)**

7) Resistance: intrinsically resistant to most antibiotics, *faecium* spp. are particularly resistant

8) Prophylaxis: hand-washing, contact isolation

B. Gram Positive Rods (GPR)

1. *Bacillus*

   a. *B. anthracis*

      1) Appearance: GPR with square ends in a chain, **appear like box-cars on a train**

      2) Lab assays: **non-motile**, spore-forming anaerobe

      3) Virulence factors:

         a) Anti-phagocytic capsule made of **D-glutamate**

         b) Anthrax toxin

            i) Tripartite toxin: protective antigen, lethal factor, and edema factor

            ii) Edema factor acts via adenylate cyclase

      4) Epidemiology: spores in soil, or on animal hide, fur, or wool transmitted via epithelial penetration or inhalation

      5) Clinical Diseases:

         a) Anthrax is a systemic sepsis syndrome characterized by a black eschar at the portal of entry, called a **"malignant pustule"**

         b) Woolsorter's disease is a severe pneumonic process caused by inhalation of spores, rapidly fatal

      6) Treatment: penicillin

      7) Resistance: none significant

      8) Prophylaxis: a moderately efficacious vaccine is available for those at high risk (e.g., abattoir workers, tanners, etc.)

   d. *B. cereus*

      1) Appearance: GPR with square ends in a chain, **appear like box-cars on a train**

      2) Lab assays: **motile**

      3) Virulence factors: exotoxins causing gastroenteritis (i.e., enterotoxin)

4) Epidemiology: spores which germinate when heated found on grains/rice

5) Clinical Diseases: gastroenteritis **classically occurs when fried rice is reheated, can occur either rapidly (within 4 hr of consumption, easily confused with *S. aureus* gastroenteritis) or after an 18-hr incubation**

6) Treatment: symptomatic support

7) Resistance: none

8) Prophylaxis: none

2. *Clostridium*

   a. *C. botulinum*

      1) Appearance: GPR with subterminal spores

      2) Lab assays: spore-forming **anaerobe**, inoculation of affected food or serum from patient causes botulism in mice

      3) Virulence factors: Botulinum toxin is preformed, inactivated by high heat-cooking, absorbed in gut, carried by bloodstream to nerve endings where it blocks the release of acetylcholine into the nerve synapse

      4) Epidemiology: spores in soil and on contaminated foods, often canned foods

      5) Clinical Diseases:

         a) Classic botulism: after ingestion of food contaminated by spores, causes classic **"descending paralysis" with significant bulbar effects** (e.g., diplopia, dysphagia) ultimately causing respiratory collapse

         b) Wound botulism: caused by contamination of wound by spores, presentation the same as classic botulism

         c) Infant botulism: **classically seen after ingestion of honey**, disease usually not fatal in infants

      6) Treatment: botulism antitoxin, respiratory support

      7) Resistance: none

      8) Prophylaxis: properly storing and cooking food, discard swollen cans

   b. *C. difficile*

1) Appearance: GPR

2) Lab assays: C-diff toxin screen in stool, anaerobic, form spores

3) Virulence factors: exotoxins cause pseudomembranous colitis, with watery/bloody diarrhea, exotoxin B ADP-ribosylates a GTP-binding protein called Rho

4) Epidemiology: transmitted fecal-orally, colonizes GI tract in up to a third of hospitalized patients, selected for by use of clindamycin (high risk of C-diff), penicillins, cephalosporins (#1 cause since they are used so frequently), and others

5) Clinical Diseases: severe gastroenteritis, with blood and mucous, can cause systemic toxicity, toxic megacolon, colonoscopy shows classic "pseudomembranes" in colon

6) Treatment: withdraw causative antibiotic, treat with oral metronidazole (1st line), or with oral vancomycin if the organism is resistant to metronidazole

7) Resistance: increasing resistance to metronidazole

8) Prophylaxis: avoid antibiotics

c. *C. perfringens*

1) Appearance: GPR, **thick**, brick-like

2) Lab assays: β-hemolytic, anaerobic, form spores

3) Virulence factors: α-toxin destroys cell membranes, other enzymes cause gas to form in tissues

4) Epidemiology: spores ubiquitous in soil, bacteria are also normal colonic and vaginal flora

5) Clinical Diseases:

    a) Gas gangrene: infects dirty wounds, classically causes **crepitation** due to subcutaneous gas, very high mortality rate from systemic shock

    b) Gastroenteritis: a self-limited infection from reheating food, **incubation period is 8–16 hr,** diarrhea is prominent but vomiting is not

6) Treatment: surgical debridement is first-line, penicillin and clindamycin are adjunctive

7) Resistance: none

8) Prophylaxis: clean wounds

d. *C. tetani*

1) Appearance: GPR, **thin,** with **terminal spores, appears like a drumstick or tennis racket**

2) Lab assays: anaerobic, form spores

3) Virulence factors: tetanus toxin is an exotoxin produced at the site of inoculation, carried by bloodstream to peripheral nerves, transported retrograde up the axon to the proximal synapse where it inhibits the release of inhibitory signals like glycine, thereby causing unopposed stimulation of the nerve

4) Epidemiology: spores ubiquitous in soil and dirty metal or glass

5) Clinical Diseases: infects dirty wounds, causing permanent neuromuscular stimulation, classic findings are **lockjaw** from inability to relax jaw muscles, and **risus sardonicus** (sardonic smile), death is ultimately secondary to respiratory failure

6) Treatment: tetanus antitoxin immunoglobulin

7) Resistance: none

8) Prophylaxis: vaccination with tetanus toxoid, a formaldehyde inactivated toxin, for particularly dirty wounds, both toxoid and immunoglobulin should be given concurrently

3. *Corynebacterium*

   a. *C. diphtheriae*

      1) Appearance: GPR, thin, **club-shaped, arranged in palisades, V- or L-shaped formations, granules stain metachromatically** (granules stain different color than the rest of the cell)

      2) Lab assays: **non-motile,** not anaerobic, do not form spores, **form black colonies on tellurite agar; Schick's test** is the injection of pure diphtheria toxin intradermally into a patient, if no inflammation occurs the patient is immune

      3) Virulence factors: diphtheria toxin ADP-ribosylates elongation factor 2 (EF-2), thereby inhibiting protein synthesis in the cell

      4) Epidemiology: transmitted from the oropharynx by respiratory droplets

      5) Clinical Diseases: diphtheria is typified by airway obstruction via formation of a **gray, fibrinous**

TABLE 4	Summary of Gram Positive Rods			
	APPEARANCE	LAB	VIRULENCE	EPIDEM.
Bacillus				
anthracis	In a chain, like box-cars	Non-motile, spore-forming anaerobe	D-glutamate capsule, tripartite toxin	Spores in soil, animal hide/fur
cereus	In a chain, like box-cars	Motile, spore-forming anaerobe	Enterotoxin	**Reheated fried rice**
Clostridium				
botulinum	Subterminal spore	Spore-forming anaerobe	Botulinum toxin blocks acetylcholine	Spores in soil and canned foods
difficile	GPR	Anaerobe, C-diff toxin in stool	C-diff toxin	Antibiotics predispose
perfringens	Thick GPR	Anaerobic, spore forming	α-toxin	Spores in soil
tetani	Thin GPR, appears like a drumstick	Anaerobic, spore forming	Tetanus toxin	Spores in soil, dirty glass or metal
Corynebacterium				
diphtheriae	Thin, palisades, metachromatic granules	Non-motile, aerobe, forms black colonies on tellurite agar: Schick's test discerns immunity or not	Diphtheria toxin	Respiratory droplets
Listeria				
monocytogenes	Tumbling motility	Motile, aerobe, β-hemolytic	Listeriolysin O	Unpasteurized dairy products

pseudomembrane in the oropharynx, myocarditis can also develop

6) Treatment: antitoxin, respiratory support

7) Resistance: none

8) Prophylaxis: diptheria toxoid, should be given to all children as part of the DTP vaccine

4. *Listeria*

   b. *L. monocytogenes*

      1) Appearance: GPR, thin, arranged in palisades, V- or L-shaped formations

      2) Lab assays: classic **tumbling motility**, not anaerobic, do not form spores, β-hemolytic

      3) Virulence factors: listeriolysin O disrupts cell membranes

      4) Epidemiology: transmitted via unpasteurized dairy products or via fecal-oral route

      5) Clinical Diseases:

         a) Neonatal meningitis or sepsis, abortion

         b) Bacteremia and meningitis occur in the immunocompromised, such as renal transplant patients, alcoholics

      6) Treatment: ampicillin +/− aminoglycoside

      7) Resistance: unusual

      8) Prophylaxis: pasteurize cheese and dairy products

C. Gram Negative Cocci (GNC)

1. *Neisseria*

   a. *N. meningitidis*

      1) Appearance: **often diplococci**, arranged like **two kidney beans** facing each other

      2) Lab assays: grow on chocolate agar (heated blood agar), oxidase positive, ferments maltose

      3) Virulence factors:

         a) Antiphagocytic capsule

         b) IgA protease

      4) Epidemiology: transmitted via respiratory droplets, colonize oropharynx, prone to outbreaks in communal settings such as college dormitory or military barracks, **people with defects in the late complement pathway (C6–C9) are prone to *Neisseria* infections**

5) Clinical Diseases:

   a) Meningitis

   b) Waterhouse–Friderichsen syndrome: sepsis resulting in DIC and adrenal failure due to adrenal gland infarction

6) Treatment: penicillin

7) Resistance: rare

8) Prophylaxis: a moderately efficacious vaccine is available for those at high risk (e.g., those in military barracks), **rifampin is used for primary prophylaxis of close contacts** of an infected patient (rifampin penetrates saliva better than penicillin, so eradicates the carrier state better)

b. *N. gonorrhoeae*

1) Appearance: often **diplococci inside neutrophils** (pathognomonic on gram stain from urethral specimen)

2) Lab assays: **growth on Thayer–Martin agar** (chocolate agar with antibiotics to suppress genitourinary colonizers), oxidase positive, does not ferment maltose

3) Virulence factors:

   a) Pili attach to mucosal surfaces

   b) Lipo-oligosaccharide (LOS) instead of lipopolysaccharide (LPS) makes the organism less stimulatory to immune cells

   c) IgA protease

4) Epidemiology: always sexually transmitted, in both males and females infection can be asymptomatic, **infections common in patients with late complement deficiencies (C6–C9)**

5) Clinical Diseases:

   a) Urethritis, pharyngitis, proctitis

   b) Pelvic inflammatory disease, salpingitis

   c) Septic arthritis

6) Treatment: ceftriaxone, fluoroquinolones 2nd line

7) Resistance: common to penicillins, due both to altered penicillin binding proteins and expression of β-lactamase

TABLE 5	**Summary of Gram Negative Cocci**			
	APPEARANCE	**LAB**	**VIRULENCE**	**EPIDEM.**
N. menin-gitidis	Diplococci, often intracellular	Oxidase positive, ferments maltose	Capsule	Communal outbreaks
N. gono-rrhoeae	Diplococci, often intracellular	Oxidase positive, does not ferment maltose, grows on Thayer–Martin media	Pili, LOS	STD, can be asymptomatic
M. cata-rrhalis	Paired coccobacillus (short rods)	Oxidase positive, does not ferment maltose	None sig.	Transmitted via respiratory droplets
Acineto-bacter	Paired coccobacillus (medium rods)	Oxidase negative	None sig.	ICU colonizer, ventilator assoc. pneumonia

8) Prophylaxis: safe sex

2. *Moraxella catarrhalis*

   1) Appearance: paired coccobacilli (rods are very short) often inside neutrophils

   2) Lab assays: oxidase positive, does not ferment maltose

   3) Virulence factors: none significant

   4) Epidemiology: respiratory droplet transmission, colonizes human oropharynx

   5) Clinical Diseases:

      a) Upper respiratory diseases: otitis/sinusitis/bronchitis

      b) Atypical pneumonia

   6) Treatment: macrolide or doxycycline

   7) Resistance: frequent β-lactamase production

   8) Prophylaxis: none

3. *Acinetobacter*

   1) Appearance: paired coccobacilli (rods are medium sized) often inside neutrophils

   2) Lab assays: oxidase negative

3) Virulence factors: none significant

4) Epidemiology: **transmission associated with pooled water, notorious ICU colonizer**

5) Clinical Diseases:

   a) **Pneumonia: always nosocomial, usually in the ICU, often in patients on ventilators**

   b) Bacteremia, secondary to pneumonia

6) Treatment: imipenem or ceftazidime plus aminoglycoside

7) Resistance: **essentially 100% β-lactamase production, extremely resistant organism,** definitive therapy depends on particular sensitivity pattern of isolate

8) Prophylaxis: contact isolation, ICU sterility

D. Gram Negative Rods (GNR)

1. Enterobacteriaceae

- A family of GNR, all are normal flora in the colon

- **All have four defining metabolic features: (1) facultative anaerobes, (2) ferment glucose, (3) oxidase negative, and (4) reduce nitrates to nitrites**

- Three classic antigens: (1) O antigen is a component of LPS in members of the Enterobacteriaceae, (2) H antigen is a flagellar protein found in *E. coli* and *Salmonella*, and (3) K antigen is a capsular polysaccharide antigen found in encapsulated organisms

- The genera are important, but individual species not important for exam purposes

a. *Escherichia coli*

   1) Appearance: GNR

   2) Lab assays: **motile,** ferments lactose as detected by forming pink colonies on MacConkey agar and green colonies on EMB agar, forms gas but not hydrogen sulfide (H_2S) on triple sugar iron (TSI) agar, **metabolizes tryptophan to indole**

   3) Virulence factors:

      a) Pili allow mucosal adhesion

      b) Enterotoxins cause watery diarrhea

    i)   Heat Stable Toxin (ST) ↑ cGMP levels in the cell, causing ion and fluid secretion

    ii) Heat Labile Toxin (LT) is almost identical to cholera toxin (see below), and ↑ cAMP

  c) **Shiga-toxin, found in *E. coli* O157:H7, causes bloody diarrhea and the hemolytic-uremic syndrome**

  d) Has O, H, and K antigens (see above)

  e) **LPS is a very potent stimulator of inflammation/sepsis**

4) Epidemiology: normal colonic flora, gastroenteritis spread by fecal-oral contact

5) Clinical Diseases:

  a) **Most common cause of UTI/pyelonephritis**

  b) Traveler's diarrhea caused by enterotoxigenic *E. coli* (ETEC)

  c) Dysentery/bloody gastroenteritis caused by enteroinvasive *E. coli* (EIEC)

  d) Hemolytic-uremic syndrome complicates gastroenteritis caused by enterohemorrhagic *E. coli* O157:H7 (EHEC), especially in children

  e) Neonatal meningitis

  f) *E. coli* bacteremia causes classic gram negative sepsis

6) Treatment: cephalosporins, Bactrim, quinolones, aminoglycosides

7) Resistance: increasing in the community to many antibiotics

8) Prophylaxis: good hygiene

b. *Salmonella*

1) Appearance: GNR

2) Lab assays: **motile**, does not ferment lactose (clear colonies on MacConkey and EMB agar), produces gas and hydrogen sulfide on TSI agar

3) Virulence factors:

  a) O, H, and K antigens

  b) *Salmonella* are subdivided by O antigens into groups A to I

4) Epidemiology: **transmitted via poultry and eggs, gastric acid is crucial to host defense, so patients on acid-reduction therapy are prone to infection, can also be transmitted by pets such as turtles, lizards, and dogs**

5) Clinical Diseases:

a) Enterocolitis: bloody gastroenteritis, typically self-limited

b) Typhoid fever: minimal GI symptoms, systemic dissemination causes fever with delirium and abdominal pain, **Rose spots** are classic rose-colored macules on the abdomen, some patients suffer intestinal perforation, during recovery *Salmonella* **colonizes the gallbladder readily and then is transmitted fecally in a carrier state (remember Typhoid Mary?)**

c) Bacteremia: can seed any organ, frequently bone in asplenic patients (e.g., sickle cell), and can cause abdominal abscesses

6) Treatment: cephalosporin, aminoglycoside, fluoroquinolone

7) Resistance: unusual

8) Prophylaxis: good hygiene

c. *Shigella*

1) Appearance: GNR

2) Lab assays: **non-motile**, does not ferment lactose (clear colonies on MacConkey and EMB agar), does not produce gas or hydrogen sulfide on TSI agar

3) Virulence factors:

a) O antigen only

b) Some strains produce Shiga-toxin

4) Epidemiology: transmitted via fecal-oral route and contaminated food, **only 100 organisms are required to establish enteric infection**

5) Clinical Diseases:

a) Enterocolitis = bloody gastroenteritis, typically self-limited

6) Treatment: supportive, fluids and electrolytes, fluoroquinolones or aminoglycosides for severe disease

7) Resistance: increasing

8) Prophylaxis: good hygiene

d. *Yersinia enterocolitica & pseudotuberculosis* (see zoonotic infections for *Y. pestis*)

1) Appearance: **oval shaped**

2) Lab assays: **non-motile at 37°C but motile at 25°C,** do not ferment lactose, do not make gas or hydrogen sulfide on TSI agar, **urease positive**

3) Virulence factors: enterotoxins

4) Epidemiology: zoonotic transmission, fecal-oral

5) Clinical Diseases:

a) Gastroenteritis with bloody diarrhea, invasive disease

b) **Mesenteric adenitis mimicking appendicitis**

6) Treatment: Bactrim or fluoroquinolones

7) Resistance: none

8) Prophylaxis: none

e. *Proteus*

1) Appearance: GNR

2) Lab assays: **motile/swarming,** does not ferment lactose, makes gas and hydrogen sulfide on TSI agar, **urease positive, phenylalanine deaminase positive**

3) Virulence factors: urease splits urea, alkalinizing urine

4) Epidemiology: causes community acquired UTIs and nosocomial infections

5) Clinical Diseases:

a) Community acquired or nosocomial UTIs

b) **Causes infected struvite stones (ammonium magnesium phosphate) via alkalinization of the urine**

c) Line sepsis

d) Bacteremia/sepsis

6) Treatment: 3rd generation cephalosporin, aminoglycoside, or fluoroquinolone

7) Resistance: increasing resistance in nosocomial infections

8) Prophylaxis: sterility during procedures and careful hand-washing

f. *Klebsiella*

1) Appearance: GNR

2) Lab assays: **non-motile,** ferments lactose, makes gas but not hydrogen sulfide on TSI agar

3) Virulence factors: large polysaccharide capsule (K antigen)

4) Epidemiology: community acquired disease affects the elderly and immunocompromised (e.g., alcoholics, diabetics, etc.), but it is also a common nosocomial pathogen

5) Clinical Diseases:

a) UTI/pyelonephritis, commonly nosocomial

b) Pneumonia, **classic "currant-jelly" sputum (thick blood), can progress to lung abscess, affects alcoholics, diabetics, and those with chronic lung disease**

c) Bacteremia/sepsis

6) Treatment: double cover with 3rd generation cephalosporin, aminoglycoside, or fluoroquinolone

7) Resistance: rapid emergence of resistance on therapy, increasing resistance in nosocomial infections

8) Prophylaxis: sterility during procedures and careful hand-washing

g. *Enterobacter*

1) Appearance: GNR

2) Lab assays: **motile,** ferments lactose, makes gas but not hydrogen sulfide on TSI agar

3) Virulence factors: none significant

4) Epidemiology: **causes nosocomial infections**

5) Clinical Diseases:

a) Line sepsis

b) UTI if catheter in place

c) Bacteremia/sepsis

d) Cholangitis

TABLE 6	Summary of Enterobacteriaceae				
	MOTILE	FERMENTS LACTOSE	TSI AGAR: GAS/H$_2$S	UNIQUE CHARACTER-ISTIC	CAUSES ENTERITIS?
E. coli	Yes	Yes	+ / −	Metabolize tryptophan to indole	Yes
Salmonella	Yes	No	+ / +	Colonize gallbladder	Yes
Shigella	No	No	− / −	Inoculum of 100 causes disease	Yes
Yersinia spp. *	Yes[#]	No	− / −	Urease ⊕	Yes
Proteus	Yes	No	+ / +	Swarming motility, urease & phenylalanine deaminase ⊕	No
Klebsiella	No	Yes	+ / −	Large polysaccharide capsule	No
Enterobacter	Yes	Yes	+ / −	Nosocomial pathogen	No
Serratia	No	No	− / −	Nosocomial pathogen	No

*Y. enterocolitica & pseudotuberculosis only, see below for *Y. pestis*;
[#]Mobile at 25°C but not 37°C

6) Treatment: aminoglycoside or fluoroquinolone or both, not ceftazadime due to extended spectrum β-lactamases (see below)

7) Resistance: **expresses extended spectrum β-lactamases (ESBL), making it resistant to all penicillin-derivatives, including ceftazidime,** resistance increasingly common

8) Prophylaxis: sterility during procedures and careful hand-washing

h. *Serratia*

1) Appearance: GNR

2) Lab assays: **non-motile,** does not ferment lactose, does not make gas or hydrogen sulfide on TSI agar

3) Virulence factors: none significant

4) Epidemiology: **causes nosocomial infections**

5) Clinical Diseases:

   a) Line sepsis

   b) UTI if catheter in place

   c) Bacteremia/sepsis

6) Treatment: 3rd generation cephalosporin, aminoglycoside, or fluoroquinolone

7) Resistance: increasing resistance in nosocomial infections

8) Prophylaxis: sterility during procedures and careful hand-washing

2. Other GNR causing enteric infections

   a. *Vibrio cholera*

      1) Appearance: GNR, **shaped like a comma (curved)**

      2) Lab assays: motile, oxidase positive, **inhibited by hypertonic saline**

      3) Virulence factors: Enterotoxin composed of two subunits, A and B

         a) Subunit A ADP-ribosylates G-protein, locking it in the stimulatory mode, resulting in overwhelming production of cAMP → secretion of chloride ion and water in the small intestine

         b) Subunit B is necessary for penetration of Subunit A into the cell

      4) Epidemiology: Fecal-oral transmission, can also be transmitted via uncooked shellfish, carriers can be asymptomatic

      5) Clinical Diseases:

         a) Watery diarrhea known as **"rice–water stool,"** no blood in the diarrhea and no abdominal pain, death is due to dehydration and electrolyte imbalance; diarrhea is secretory, originates in the small intestine

      6) Treatment: **Oral rehydration with salt solution, glucose must be included in the rehydration solution to**

increase ion uptake in the gut via the sodium–glucose cotransporter; antibiotics not indicated

7) Resistance: none

8) Prophylaxis: good hygiene and public health efforts

b. *Vibrio parahaemolyticus*

1) Appearance: GNR, **shaped like a comma (curved)**

2) Lab assays: motile, oxidase positive, **resistant to hypertonic saline**

3) Virulence factors: Enterotoxin similar to *V. cholera*

4) Epidemiology: **The bacteria lives in the ocean, typically transmitted by uncooked fish** (common cause of diarrhea in Japan and on cruise ships)

5) Clinical Diseases:

   a) Diarrhea of variable severity, typically self-limited, diarrhea is caused by enteroinvasion of colon and can sometimes be bloody

6) Treatment: supportive

7) Resistance: none

8) Prophylaxis: adequately cooking seafood

c. *Vibrio vulnificus*

1) Appearance: GNR, **shaped like a comma (curved)**

2) Lab assays: motile, oxidase positive, **resistant to hypertonic saline**

3) Virulence factors: none significant

4) Epidemiology: Like *V. parahaemolyticus*, **V. vulnificus also lives in the ocean, typically transmitted via contact with fresh shellfish**

5) Clinical Diseases:

   a) **Cellulitis in fishermen/shellfish handlers**

   b) **Severe sepsis in patients with cirrhosis** or other chronic diseases who ingest raw shellfish infected with the organism

6) Treatment: 3rd generation cephalosporin +/– doxycycline or fluoroquinolone

7) Resistance: poorly characterized

8) Prophylaxis: adequately cooking seafood

d. *Campylobacter jejuni*

1) Appearance: GNR, **shaped like an "S"**

2) Lab assays: motile, oxidase positive, **microaerophilic** (grows better in 5% O_2 than 20%), urease negative

3) Virulence factors: can produce a cholera-like toxin

4) Epidemiology: Fecal-oral transmission, transmitted via domesticated animals

5) Clinical Diseases:

   a) **Most common cause of bacterial gastroenteritis in the US**, the organism is invasive so blood and mucous are typically found in the stool

6) Treatment: fluoroquinolone

7) Resistance: increasing, even to quinolones

8) Prophylaxis: adequately cooking seafood

e. *Helicobacter pylori*

1) Appearance: GNR, **shaped like an "S"**

2) Lab assays: motile, oxidase positive, **urease positive**

3) Virulence factors: urease

4) Epidemiology: Likely fecal-oral transmission

5) Clinical Diseases: gastric/duodenal ulcers, gastric carcinoma and lymphoma are associated with *H. pylori*, and **treating *H. pylori* can make some lymphomas regress**

6) Treatment: Triple Tx = amoxicillin + clarithromycin + omeprazole (other regimens available as well)

7) Resistance: increasing

8) Prophylaxis: none

f. *Bacteroides fragilis*

1) Appearance: GNR

2) Lab assays: **strict anaerobe, non-spore forming**

3) Virulence factors: antiphagocytic polysaccharide capsule

4) Epidemiology: **most common bacteria in the intestines**, about 10^{11} per gram of feces, infections are

TABLE 7 Summary of Enteric GNR			
	SHAPE	**LAB**	**HABITAT**
Vibrio cholera	Comma	Inhibited by hypertonic saline	Human host
Vibrio parahaemolyticus	Comma	**Resistant to hypertonic saline**	Ocean
Vibrio vulnificus	Comma	**Resistant to hypertonic saline**	Ocean
Campylobacter jejuni	Like an "S"	Microaerophilic, urease negative	Domestic animals
Helicobacter pylori	Like an "S"	**Urease positive**	Human host
Bacteroides fragilis	GNR	**Strict anaerobe**	Human colon

all endogenous due to translocation of *Bacteroides* across a break in the intestinal mucosa

5) Clinical Diseases: Participates in polymicrobial abscesses, peritonitis, and sepsis following disruption of bowel

6) Treatment: metronidazole 1st line, clindamycin and cefotetan are 2nd line

7) Resistance: none to metronidazole, express β-lactamase

8) Prophylaxis: none

3. GNR causing respiratory infections

   a. *Hemophilus influenza*

      1) Appearance: cocco-bacillus (can be confused with cocci)

      2) Lab assays: Growth on chocolate agar requires supplementation with **Factor V (NAD) and Factor X (heme), quellung reaction positive**

      3) Virulence factors:

         a) Polysaccharide capsule allows identification of six serotypes, **of which type b is the most virulent due to its unique polyribitol phosphate capsule structure**

         b) IgA protease

4) Epidemiology: Respiratory transmission, used to be the most common cause of meningitis but now is rare due to childhood vaccination

5) Clinical Diseases:

   a) Community acquired pneumonia

   b) Bronchitis/sinusitis/otitis media

   c) Meningitis: **95% due to serotype b**, usually occurs between ages of 6 months to 2 years, after maternal IgG levels decline and before endogenous antibody is produced against the capsule

   d) In small children epiglottitis can occur, which is a medical emergency due to risk of laryngospasm causing respiratory arrest, presents with quiet/still child leaning forward and drooling due to inability to swallow, has classic "thumb" sign on lateral neck x-rays

6) Treatment: meningitis requires 3rd generation cephalosporin, treat upper respiratory infections with amoxicillin or Bactrim, treat pneumonia with 3rd generation cephalosporins or macrolides

7) Resistance: many strains produce β-lactamase

8) Prophylaxis:

   a) Extremely effective vaccine—**due to inability of small children to make specific antibodies directed at polysaccharide, the vaccine is a fusion of *H. influenza* polysaccharide linked to a carrier protein**

   b) Use rifampin for close contact prophylaxis for patients with meningitis

b. *Legionella pneumophila*

   1) Appearance: Gram stains faintly, hard to see

   2) Lab assays: **classically, sputum gram stain shows neutrophils but no bacteria** (because they stain poorly), **require iron and cysteine supplementation to grow in culture**

   3) Virulence factors: none significant

   4) Epidemiology: Infectious outbreaks **associated with contaminated sources of water** (e.g., air conditioners, sinks, showers), although infections are transmitted via

the lung, **person-to-person spread does not occur, most patients with severe disease are elderly, smoke, drink, or have a cell-mediated immune defect** (e.g., HIV, treated with steroids, renal transplant)

5) Clinical Diseases:

a) Pontiac fever: mild flu-like illness

b) Severe multilobar pneumonia with systemic toxicity, **commonly associated with diarrhea** (always think *Legionella* in a patient with pneumonia and diarrhea), **very high LDH, pulse-fever dissociation, and hyponatremia**

6) Treatment: 2nd generation macrolide (e.g., clarithromycin or azithromycin) and fluoroquinolones are both first line

7) Resistance: frequently produce β-lactamases

8) Prophylaxis: avoid contaminated water

c. *Bordetella pertussis*

1) Appearance: small cocco-bacillus

2) Lab assays: Growth requires **Bordet-Gengou agar**

3) Virulence factors:

a) Pili allow attachment to respiratory epithelia

b) Pertussis toxin: **ADP-ribosylates an inhibitory G-protein**, blocking its activity, thereby allowing unopposed stimulation of adenylate cyclase → **high cAMP production** (contrast this with cholera toxin, which also stimulates high cAMP production but does so by ADP-ribosylating a stimulatory G-protein, thereby locking it into active form)

4) Epidemiology: Highly contagious, transmitted by respiratory droplets, severe disease is rare in the developed world due to widespread vaccination, but it can cause chronic cough in adults

5) Clinical Diseases:

a) **Whooping cough: tracheobronchitis** affecting children, begins with a week of mild respiratory symptoms, followed by paroxysmal coughing attacks lasting up to 4 weeks (**the "whoop" is the characteristic sound made during the gasp for inhalation after a spasm of coughing**), pronounced lymphocytosis can occur

b) A flu-like illness or chronic cough can occur in adults whose immunity has waned

6) Treatment: supportive, macrolides to shorten duration

7) Resistance: none

8) Prophylaxis: both whole cell, killed vaccine (part of DPT) and an acellular vaccine are in widespread use

d. *Pseudomonas aeruginosa*

1) Appearance: GNR

2) Lab assays: strict aerobe, oxidase positive, does not ferment glucose (in contrast to Enterobacteriaceae), does not ferment lactose (clear colonies on MacConkey or EMB agar), secretes pyocyanin and pyoverdin, which cause agar to become blue-green colored around a colony, **causes a fruity smell**, does not form gas or H_2S on TSI agar

3) Virulence factors:

a) Glycocalyx slime prevents phagocytosis

b) Exotoxin A works like diphtheria toxin, ADP-ribosylates EF-2, preventing protein synthesis

4) Epidemiology: common environmental water colonizer, rarely colonizes human colon, is fastidious and can survive disinfectants, as a result **is a major nosocomial pathogen**

5) Clinical Diseases:

a) **Nosocomial infections**: UTI, pneumonia, bacteremia

b) Commonly infects burns or open wounds

c) Hot-tub cellulitis

d) **Malignant otitis externa in diabetics**

e) **Recurrent pneumonia in cystic fibrosis patients**

6) Treatment: **double cover** with a combination of ceftazidime, extended spectrum penicillin with β-lactamase inhibitor (e.g., piperacillin/tazobactam), aminoglycoside, or ciprofloxacin

7) Resistance: highly resistant to multiple antibiotics, and new **resistance occurs quickly on single therapy, so always double cover for severe disease**

8) Prophylaxis: hand-washing, sterility during procedures

TABLE 8	Summary of Respiratory GNR	
ORGANISM	**LAB**	**INFECTIONS**
Hemophilus	Factor V (NAD) & Factor X (heme) required for growth, quellung reaction ⊕	Rare now due to vaccine
Legionella	Iron & cysteine required for growth, gram stain shows multiple neutrophils but no bacteria (stain poorly)	Water is the source; Diarrhea, ⇑LDH, pulse-fever dissociation, & hyponatremia commonly seen
Bordetella	Grow on Bordet–Gengou agar	Very contagious
Pseudomonas	Agar turns green due to pyocyanin & pyoverdin, causes a fruity smell	Nosocomial pathogen, highly antibiotic resistant

4. GNR causing zoonotic infections

   a. *Bartonella henselae & quintana*

      1) Appearance: small coccobacillus

      2) Lab assays: diagnosis made by serology or biopsy

      3) Virulence factors: none significant

      4) Epidemiology: **body louse is proven to transmit B. quintana, B. henselae can be transmitted by cat scratches (particularly kittens) and also possibly by body louse or fleas,** *B. quintana* is associated with poor sanitation and cramped conditions such as refugee camps or trenches during war, while *B. henselae* is associated with homelessness

      5) Clinical Diseases:

         a) Cat-scratch disease: caused by *B. henselae*, presents with constitutional symptoms (e.g., fevers, chills, night-sweats), and diffuse, **massive lymphadenopathy affecting nodes nearest inoculation** (e.g., if scratch is on forearm nodes, extend up the arm to the axilla), can mimic lymphoma

         b) Bacillary angiomatosis: also caused by *B. henselae*, **a disseminated disease typically seen in AIDS patients,** bacteremia with fevers, chills, myalgias, and **characteristic red nodules all over the body**

composed of small capillary hemangiomas which can appear like Kaposi's sarcoma

c) Trench fever: caused by *B. quintana*, transmitted by body louse, presents with abrupt onset high fevers, chills, myalgias, can cause multiple paroxysms of fever separated by afebrile periods

6) Treatment: doxycycline or macrolides

7) Resistance: none

8) Prophylaxis: good hygiene, avoid scratches by kittens

b. *Brucella*

1) Appearance: small coccobacillus

2) Lab assays: diagnosis made by serology

3) Virulence factors: none significant

4) Epidemiology: **transmitted via contaminated milk or via direct contact with sheep, pigs, or cattle**

5) Clinical Diseases:

d) **Undulating fever: mono-like illness with constitutional symptoms, hepatosplenomegaly and diffuse adenopathy, fever waxes and wanes daily**

6) Treatment: doxycycline plus aminoglycoside

7) Resistance: none

8) Prophylaxis: pasteurize milk

c. *Francisella tularensis*

1) Appearance: small coccobacillus

2) Lab assays: not cultured in lab due to risk of inhalational infection, diagnosis made by DFA or agglutination

3) Virulence factors: none significant

4) Epidemiology: typical host is rabbit or vermin, **usually transmitted by tick (also by lice or mite)**

5) Clinical Diseases:

a) Multiple forms of disease, most common is "ulcero-glandular" type, an ulceration occurs at the site of inoculation, and diffuse lymphadenopathy develops, causing mono-like illness, can also cause pneumonia

      6) Treatment: streptomycin is 1st line (the only remaining disease for which streptomycin is 1st line), alternative is any aminoglycoside

      7) Resistance: none

      8) Prophylaxis: live attenuated vaccine, moderately effective, given to people whose occupation places them at high risk (e.g., tanner, fur-trapper)

  d. *Pasteurella multocida*

      1) Appearance: small coccobacillus, **bipolar staining** (like a safety pin, the ends stain but clear in the middle)

      2) Lab assays: none helpful, diagnosis is presumptive/clinical

      3) Virulence factors: antiphagocytic capsule

      4) Epidemiology: **inoculated during dog or cat bites**, part of a polymicrobial cellulitis

      5) Clinical Diseases: **dog- or cat-bite cellulitis**

      6) Treatment: amoxicillin/clavulonic acid for polymicrobial infection

      7) Resistance: unusual

      8) Prophylaxis: animal bites should not be sutured to prevent abscess formation

  e. *Yersinia pestis*

      1) Appearance: small coccobacillus, **bipolar staining** (like a safety pin, the ends stain but clear in the middle)

      2) Lab assays: great care must be taken during culturing to prevent airborne infection in the lab

      3) Virulence factors: antiphagocytic capsule

      4) Epidemiology: majority of cases in the world occur in SE Asia, but plague is endemic in the western US, host is vermin, vector is flea, person to person transmission also occurs via respiratory droplets

      5) Clinical Diseases:

         a) Bubonic plague: **painful swelling of lymph nodes known as bubo typifies disease**, eventually the bubo ulcerates, within days the disease progresses to systemic toxicity, including severe pneumonia, DIC, sepsis/shock, **50% lethal without treatment**

TABLE 9	Summary of Zoonotic GNR	
ORGANISM	**DISEASE CHARACTERISTICS**	**EPIDEMIOLOGY**
Bartonella henselae	Cat-scratch dz causes lymphadenopathy. Bacillary angiomatosis causes diffuse skin hemangiomas	Cat-scratch transmitted by kittens. Bacillary angiomatosis typically seen in AIDS patients
Bartonella quintana	Trench fever with abrupt onset fever, can be paroxysmal	Seen in crowded, unsanitary conditions, associated with war and homelessness
Brucella	Undulating fever = waxes and wanes over weeks to months	Transmitted via dairy products, or contact with sheep, pigs, or cattle
Francisella	Ulceroglandular = ulcer forms at site of inoculation, diffuse adenopathy	Rabbit or vermin are host, vector is tick
Pasteurella	Cellulitis from dog or cat bites	Presumptive from dog or cat bites
Yersinia pestis	Buboes	Vermin are hosts, flea is vector

    b) Pneumonic plague: **inhalation of contaminated respiratory droplets, much more rapid systemic course, 100% lethal without treatment**

6) Treatment: high dose gentamicin, treat preemptively, do NOT wait for gram stain or culture results

7) Resistance: none

8) Prophylaxis: vermin control, flea control, quarantine infected patients

E. Atypical Bacteria (Gram Stain Unrevealing)

1. Acid Fast Bacteria

   a. *Actinomyces*

     1) Appearance: long, **filamentous** bacteria, **weakly acid fast and also weakly gram positive**

     2) Lab assays: anaerobic, **"sulfur granules"** are yellowish crystalloid-appearing clumps which are revealed to be clumped organisms when seen under microscope

3) Virulence factors: none significant

4) Epidemiology: normal flora of human oropharynx

5) Clinical Diseases: can cause abscesses and invasive infections in any organ, typically seen in head and neck or in abdomen, dental infections common, **readily crosses tissue planes and erodes through bones, causing sinus tracts that drain from organs through the skin—"sinus tract" and "sulfur granules" are the key words to look for on an exam**

6) Treatment: penicillin and surgical debridement

7) Resistance: none

8) Prophylaxis: none

b. *Mycobacterium avium-intracellulare*

1) Appearance: acid fast bacilli

2) Lab assays: cultures require up to 3 weeks to grow

3) Virulence factors: none significant

4) Epidemiology: ubiquitous in the environment, **disease develops in AIDS patients when CD4 count drops below 50**

5) Clinical Diseases:

a) Disseminated disease: more common than pulmonary disease, causes fevers, weight loss, **lymphadenopathy, bone marrow suppression (pancytopenia)**, and chronic gastroenteritis, seen when CD4 is less than 50

b) Pulmonary disease: relatively rare, indistinguishable from TB clinically

6) Treatment: Multiple drug regimen, always include 2nd generation macrolide (clarithromycin or azithromycin) as cornerstone, as well as ethambutol

7) Resistance: uncommon

8) Prophylaxis: all AIDS patients with CD4 counts less than 50 should receive azithromycin prophylaxis once per week

c. *Mycobacteria leprae*

1) Appearance: acid fast bacilli seen within **foamy macrophages** (lipid laden) on biopsy

2) Lab assays: obligate aerobe, cannot grow in culture, **must grow in armadillo footpads,** prefers growth at 30°C

3) Virulence factors: none significant

4) Epidemiology: transmitted by **prolonged** contact with secretions or skin of infected person

5) Clinical Diseases:

    a) **Lepromatous leprosy: the disseminated form seen in patients with poor cell-mediated immune responses to the organism,** the bacteria disseminates and grows uncontrolled in peripheral nerve endings, fingers, and earlobes (sites where body temperature is lower than core temperature)

    b) **Tuberculoid leprosy: strong delayed type hypersensitivity consistent with potent cell-mediated immunity, typified by relative control of disease with diminished organism burden on biopsy**

6) Treatment: dapsone plus rifampin for up to 2 years

7) Resistance: prone to resistance without dual therapy

8) Prophylaxis: consider dapsone for close contacts

d. *Mycobacterium marinarum*

1) Appearance: acid fast bacilli

2) Lab assays: **photochromogenic = forms yellow pigment when exposed to light**

3) Virulence factors: none significant

4) Epidemiology: lives in fresh water (e.g., fish tank, swimming pool)

5) Clinical Diseases: **"Fish-tank granuloma," infection develops after minor trauma causes break in skin with subsequent exposure of skin to fresh water environments,** results in progressive ulceration with heaped up borders

6) Treatment: 2nd generation macrolide (clarithromycin or azithromycin) or doxycycline

7) Resistance: none

8) Prophylaxis: avoid skin breaks

e. *Mycobacterium tuberculosis*

1) Appearance: cords of **acid fast bacilli**, stain red on Ziehl-Neelsen prep due to high cell wall content of mycolic acids

2) Lab assays: obligate aerobe, requires Lowenstein-Jensen medium for growth, doubling time = 18 hours (versus 20 minutes for *E. coli*) **so can take up to 8 weeks for cultures to grow, TB is the only *Mycobacterium* that produces niacin**

3) Virulence factors: cord factor allows growth in extended chains

4) Epidemiology: exposure is by respiratory droplets; however, **only 3% of exposed patients develop active disease per year, risk of active disease is increased by depressed immune status** (e.g., elderly, HIV+, malnourished, etc.)

5) Clinical Diseases:

   a) Pulmonary TB: **primary disease occurs in the lung bases, reactivation disease occurs in the upper lobes** due to higher oxygen tension which supports the organism better, disease course typified by chronic cough, hemoptysis, fevers, night sweats, weight loss, lymphadenopathy—**look for Ghon complex on CXR,** which is a granuloma with an adjacent calcified lymph node

   b) TB can disseminate to any organ

6) Treatment: four drug therapy = RIPE (rifampin, isoniazid, pyrazinamide, ethambutol) × 2 months, subsequently narrow to 2 drug therapy (isoniazid, rifampin) for a total of 6 months to 1 year of treatment (up to 2 years in HIV+ patients)

7) Resistance: increasingly common, multi-drug resistant (MDR) TB is of particular concern

8) Prophylaxis: based upon PPD test

   a) Purified Protein Derivative, administered intradermally, **useful as a screening test in asymptomatic patients but is NOT useful as a diagnostic test in symptomatic patients**

   b) New guidelines from 2000 recommend to prophylax *all* people with positive PPD regardless of age but to only put PPDs on people whom it is safe to prophylax (e.g., don't put a PPD on a low risk person >35 yr old)

TABLE 10	Summary of Acid Fast Bacilli	
ORGANISM	**APPEARANCE**	**DISEASE CHARACTERISTICS**
Actinomyces	Filamentous, weakly gram positive & acid fast	Look for "sulfur granules," organism causes draining sinus tracts and crosses tissue planes
M. avium intracellulare	Indistinguishable from TB by microscopy	Suspect in AIDS or cancer patient with pancytopenia and lymphadenopathy
M. leprae	AFBs in foamy macrophages	Organism grows in cool spots of body, e.g., ear lobes, nose, fingers, peripheral nerves
M. marinarum	Forms yellow pigment when exposed to light	"Fish-tank" granuloma, occurs following skin break and fresh water exposure
M. tuberculosis	AFBs in cords (chains)	Primary lung disease at bases, reactivation occurs at apices, look for Ghon complex = granuloma + calcified lymph node on CXR
Nocardia	Filamentous, do not gram stain	Lung disease most common, look for eosinophilia

i) 15 mm is positive in a healthy, asymptomatic person **without risk of exposure**

ii) 10 mm is positive in an asymptomatic patient **with risks**, including **immigrant** from a high risk area (e.g., SE Asia, Central/South America), pt from a medically underserved population (e.g., **homeless**), pt with a history of recent **imprison-ment**, pt **exposed to high risk individuals** (e.g., **health care workers** like us, **immigration officers**, etc.)

iii) 5 mm is positive in "high risk" pts, such as asymptomatic pt with **known exposure** to someone with active disease or pt with **debili-tating illness**, including **HIV**, **malignancy** of any kind, **cirrhosis**, **renal failure**, etc., or with CXR consistent with old disease

iv) One-third of people with active pulmonary disease have negative PPDs with positive control (specifically anergic to TB) and 50% of people with disseminated disease have negative PPDs with positive control—**therefore PPD should NOT be used as a diagnostic test in someone with symptoms of active disease**

b) **Prophylax all patients for 9 months regardless of HIV status (new guidelines from 2000)**

c) BCG vaccine is a live attenuated strain of *M. bovis* which shows some cross-protection to TB, but due to modest efficacy, short duration of protection, and invariable false-positive PPD seen after vaccination, it is not used in the US

f. *Nocardia*

1) Appearance: thin **filaments or rods, acid fast and do not gram stain** (see Figure 1)

2) Lab assays: **aerobic, can cause an eosinophilia**

3) Virulence factors: none significant

4) Epidemiology: ubiquitous in environment, causes disease in immunocompromised

5) Clinical Diseases: typically starts as pneumonia, but can disseminate especially to brain or kidneys, **mimics TB**

6) Treatment: Bactrim and surgical debridement

7) Resistance: occasional

8) Prophylaxis: none

2. Bacteria Not Seen with Gram Stain or Acid Fast

a. *Chlamydia spp.*

1) Appearance: form intracellular inclusion bodies, cannot be seen outside host cell

2) Lab assays: all are obligate intracellular parasites, and cannot be grown on media, have complex life cycle including extracellular elementary body which is like a spore, and the intracellular reticulate body which is like a germinative form which undergoes fission to produce daughter elementary bodies, **seen as inclusion bodies inside cell**

3) Virulence factors: none significant

4) Epidemiology: *C. pneumonia* transmitted via respiratory droplets, *C. psittaci* transmitted via inhalation of bird feces, *C. trachomatis* transmitted via sexual contact or

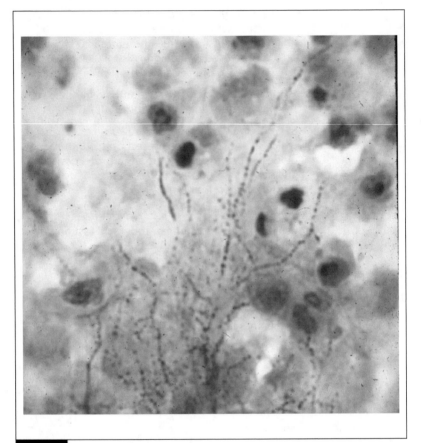

FIGURE 1

*The typical microscopic appearance of **Nocardia** in tissue, with long, thin, beaded, filamentous-like structures. Actinomyces appears similarly.*

vertically at birth, and causes eye disease by direct finger/fomite to eye contact

5) Clinical Diseases:

    a) *C. pneumonia*

        i) Upper respiratory infections: otitis, sinusitis, bronchitis

        ii) Atypical pneumonia: nagging, non-productive, cough

    b) *C. psittaci* causes Psittacosis, pneumonia, high fever, headache

c) *C. trachomatis*

    i)   Serotypes A–C cause **trachoma**: chronic conjunctivitis leading to scarring blindness over years, **this is the leading cause of blindness worldwide**

    ii) Serotypes D–K cause GU infections: urethritis, prostatitis, cervicitis, pelvic inflammatory disease

    iii) Serotypes L1–L3 cause **lymphogranuloma venereum**: STD with large inguinal adenopathy causing the **groove sign** = groove of skin between two swollen lymph nodes

6) Treatment: macrolides or doxycycline, fluoroquinolones

7) Resistance: none

8) Prophylaxis: personal hygiene, safe sex

b. *Coxiella burnetii*

1) Appearance: can't be seen by light microscopy

2) Lab assays: obligate intracellular parasite, diagnosed by serology

3) Virulence factors: none significant

4) Epidemiology: transmitted via aerosolized particulates **from exposure to farm animals like cattle, sheep, and goats, especially to products of conception (e.g., placenta)**

5) Clinical Diseases: Q fever = flu-like illness with fever and **particularly intense headache, and a classic combination of pneumonia and hepatitis,** rash is distinctly unusual

6) Treatment: doxycycline

7) Resistance: none

8) Prophylaxis: avoid products of conception of farm animals

c. *Ehrlichia*

1) Appearance: seen as intracellular inclusions in granulocytes (human granulocytic ehrlichiosis) or monocytes (human monocytic ehrlichiosis)

2) Lab assays: serologies

3) Virulence factors: none significant

4) Epidemiology: transmitted by ticks in rural areas in the south and east coast of the US

5) Clinical Diseases:

a) Human granulocytic ehrlichiosis and human monocytic ehrlichiosis have similar presentations, with fevers, chills, myalgias, occasional maculopapular rash, and **a classic triad of leukopenia, thrombocytopenia, and transaminitis,** CNS disease can occur:

6) Treatment: doxycycline

7) Resistance: none

8) Prophylaxis: avoid tick exposures

d. *Mycoplasma pneumonia*

1) Appearance: Smallest bacteria, 0.3 μm in diameter, **lack cell walls so cannot be seen on gram stain,** in culture colonies take on classic **"fried egg"** appearance with thick center colony and flatter circular edge

2) Lab assays: must culture on media containing cholesterol because *Mycoplasma* **are the only bacteria that contain cholesterol in their cell membrane; cold agglutinins** are IgM antibodies which form against the organism, and cause red blood cell agglutination, a convenient diagnostic test

3) Virulence factors: none significant

4) Epidemiology: transmitted via respiratory droplets

5) Clinical Diseases:

a) Upper respiratory infections: otitis/sinusitis/bronchitis

b) **Walking pneumonia:** most commonly affects **teens and young adults,** classic scenario is college dormitory or military barracks, subacute onset over 2–4 weeks of increasingly severe, **nagging, non-productive cough, severity of disease seen on CXR is out of proportion to mild symptoms,** disease is self-limiting in most cases

6) Treatment: macrolide or doxycycline, cell wall inhibitors (e.g., penicillins and cephalosporins) are useless since *Mycoplasma* has no cell wall

7) Resistance: none

8) Prophylaxis: none

TABLE 11	Summary of Intracellular Atypical Pathogens	
ORGANISM	**LAB**	**CHARACTERISTICS**
Chlamydia spp.	Inclusion bodies inside cells	Atypical pneumonia, conjunctivitis, or STD
Coxiella	Serology	Severe headache, pneumonia, hepatitis
Ehrlichia	Serology	Leukopenia, thrombocytopenia, transaminitis
Mycoplasma	"fried egg" colony morphology, cold agglutinins positive	Walking pneumonia seen in college-aged people, nagging cough with CXR out of proportion to symptoms
Rickettsia spp.	Weil–Felix test positive	Rocky Mountain Spotted Fever → petechial rash starting on hands and feet and moving to trunk—Typhus → petechial rash starting on trunk and moving to hands and feet

    e. *Rickettsia spp.*

       1) Appearance: tiny rods, do not gram stain

       2) Lab assays: all are obligate intracellular parasites, **Weil–Felix test detects *Rickettsia* by cross-reaction of anti-*Rickettsial* antibodies to the O-antigen of *Proteus spp.***

       3) Virulence factors: none significant

       4) Epidemiology: all are transmitted via bite of arthropods (ticks, fleas, lice)

       5) Clinical Diseases:

          a) **Rocky Mountain Spotted Fever:** caused by *R. rickettsii* **transmitted by tick, occurs on east coast of US** (not Rocky Mountain states), causes systemic vasculitis with fevers, myalgias, headache, **petechial rash starts on hands and feet and moves in to trunk**, DIC and shock can occur

          b) **Typhus:** scrub typhus transmitted via chiggers, endemic typhus via fleas, epidemic typhus via lice, starts with flu-like symptoms, **petechial rash starts on trunk and moves outward to hands and feet,** vasculitis causes CNS alterations and shock

6) Treatment: doxycycline

7) Resistance: none

8) Prophylaxis: reduction in arthropod populations

3. Spirochetal organisms

a. *Treponema pallidum* (Syphilis)

1) Appearance: poorly visualized by light microscopy, can visualize by **dark-field microscopy**

2) Lab assays: cannot be grown in culture, detect by serologies

a) RPR/VDRL

i) Detect antibodies to host phospholipids that cross-react to *Treponema* cell surface

ii) 80% positive in primary disease, 100% in secondary disease, 85% in tertiary disease

iii) Serology positive acutely but becomes negative with treatment/remission

iv) **False positives with lupus or other chronic inflammatory diseases**

b) FTA-ABS

i) Antibody directly detects *Treponemal* antigen

ii) **100% positive in secondary disease, 95% in tertiary disease**

iii) Positive for life after first exposure, so cannot distinguish between old/treated disease and re-infection

iv) **Highly specific, minimal false-positive**

3) Virulence factors: none significant

4) Epidemiology: transmitted directly through intact skin or via sexual contact

5) Clinical Diseases:

a) Primary disease: **chancre = painless ulcer** at site of inoculation, sometimes accompanied by local adenopathy, ulcer heals spontaneously

b) Secondary disease: almost all untreated patients progress to secondary stage, with **diffuse maculopapular rash that affects palms and soles** (most rashes don't), and development of **moist genital warts called condyloma lata,** bacteremia results in widespread organ seeding including liver/spleen and meninges

c) Latent syphilis

   i) One-third of patients spontaneously cure without treatment after secondary disease, 2/3 progress to latent syphilis

   ii) Early latent syphilis is marked by one or more relapses of secondary disease for several years

   iii) Late latent syphilis is asymptomatic persistent disease, develops in 50% of those with early latent syphilis, progresses to tertiary disease

d) Tertiary syphilis

   i) **Develops in 1/3 of those initially infected** (2/3 of initially infected get secondary disease, 50% of whom progress to tertiary syphilis)

   ii) **Causes gummas** (erosive ulcerations of bone, skin, or soft tissue), **tabes dorsalis, dementia paralytica, aortitis**

e) Congenital syphilis: **transmitted transplacentally only after the first trimester, causes snuffles** (bloody nasal discharge), **saber shins, Hutchinson teeth** (notched incisors), **saddle nose**

6) Treatment: penicillin G or ceftriaxone, **watch out for Jarisch–Herxheimer reaction,** which is rigors and flu-like symptoms after first dose of antibiotics (hypersensitivity reaction to antigens released by bacterial lysis)

7) Resistance: none

8) Prophylaxis: safe sex

b. *Borrelia burgdorferi*

1) Appearance: visualize by dark-field microscopy or Wright–Giemsa stain

2) Lab assays: difficult to diagnose, serology and PCR utilized

3) Virulence factors: none significant

4) Epidemiology: transmitted via tick bite (*Ixodes scapularis*), endemic to New England area, also more

rarely occurs in mountainous areas of California, usually occurs in summer

5) Clinical Diseases: Lyme disease: starts with erythema chronicum migrans, a spreading bulls-eye rash, within months progresses to myocarditis with heart block, meningitis, and cranial nerve palsies (Bell's is common), over years severe arthritis and dementia/CNS changes occur

6) Treatment: doxycycline or ceftriaxone

7) Resistance: none

8) Prophylaxis: tick repellent, wear long-sleeves and pants in wooded areas, there are now two vaccines available with good efficacy short-term (long-term not yet known), should be given to people in high-risk areas

c. *Borrelia recurrentis/hermsii*

1) Appearance: visualize by **dark-field microscopy** or Wright–Giemsa stain

2) Lab assays: diagnose by Wright–Giemsa stain of blood

3) Virulence factors: **antigen phase variation**, due to DNA cassette switching of genes coding for outer membrane antigens, allows the organism to stay one step ahead of the antibody response directed at any one antigen

4) Epidemiology: transmitted via tick or body louse

5) Clinical Diseases: **Relapsing fever**: causes flu-like illness with lymphadenopathy that lasts for several weeks, then goes away for several weeks, then recurs multiple times (resolution occurs when antibody response catches up to antigen variation, then the organism switches antigen again and the disease relapses)

6) Treatment: doxycycline

7) Resistance: none

8) Prophylaxis: tick repellent, wear long-sleeves and pants in wooded areas

d. *Leptospira*

1) Appearance: visualize by **dark-field microscopy**

2) Lab assays: difficult to diagnose, can use serologies

3) Virulence factors: none significant

TABLE 12	Summary of Spirochetes	
ORGANISM	**LAB**	**CHARACTERISTICS**
Treponema pallidum	RPR/VDRL for acute disease, FTA is more specific but cannot distinguish acute from old disease	1°dz = chancre; 2°dz = maculopapular rash on palms & soles; 3°dz = gummas, aortitis, CNS dz
Borrelia burgdorferi	Organism may be seen in peripheral blood by Wright–Giemsa stain	Bulls-eye rash, myocarditis, arthritis, CNS/PNS disease
B. recurrentis/ hermsii	Organism may be seen in peripheral blood by Wright–Giemsa stain	Recurrent fever alternating with asymptomatic periods
Leptospira	Serology may be helpful	Exposure to animal urine, biphasic illness with hepatitis, renal failure and meningitis

4) Epidemiology: **transmitted via rat, dog, or cat urine**, organism lives in fresh water, **typical case scenario is people swimming in lake in wilderness area**

5) Clinical Diseases: **Weil's Disease (icterohemorrhagic fever) relapsing fever**: a **biphasic illness** starting with flu-like symptoms followed by resolution for a few days, and then a second phase with diffuse organ involvement, including **hepatitis, acute renal failure, and aseptic meningitis**

6) Treatment: penicillin

7) Resistance: none

8) Prophylaxis: avoid rat, cat, dog, urine—better yet, avoid urine in general!

III. FUNGI

A. Yeast & Dimorphic Fungi

1. Cutaneous & Subcutaneous Pathogens

   a. *Malassezia furfur* AKA *Pityrosporum ovale*

      1) Appearance: KOH prep of skin lesions show yeast and short hyphae

TABLE 13	Summary of Cutaneous Yeast	
ORGANISM	**LAB**	**CHARACTERISTICS**
Malassezia furfur	Lesions fluoresce yellow-green under Woods lamp	Hypopigmented macules in dark-skinned people, hyperpigmented macules in light-skinned people
Sporothrix schenckii	Cigar-shaped yeast on KOH prep	Inoculated by thorn puncturing skin, look for nodules sprouting up in a line along the lymphatics of the arm

2) Lab assays: **fluoresces yellow-green under Woods lamp** (shine the lamp right on the patient's skin, over the macular skin lesions)

3) Virulence factors: none significant

4) Epidemiology: ubiquitous, particularly in tropics, transmitted by direct contact or fomites

5) Clinical Diseases: Tinea versicolor: multiple spherical macules, usually distributed on trunk; **in dark-skinned people the lesions are hypopigmented, in light-skinned people they can be hyperpigmented**

6) Treatment: topical azole cream

7) Resistance: none

8) Prophylaxis: none

b. *Sporothrix schenckii*

1) Appearance: KOH prep of skin lesions show **cigar-shaped budding yeast**

2) Lab assays: in culture at <37°C it grows as a mold, but converts to oval yeast at 37°C

3) Virulence factors: none significant

4) Epidemiology: ubiquitous on plants, infection requires antecedent trauma to disrupt the skin barrier, and the **classic scenario (especially on the boards) is infection in a gardener working with rose bushes or anyone suffering a thorn puncture wound**

5) Clinical Diseases: Sporotrichosis: local nodule forms at the site of inoculation which may ulcerate, and **additional nodules sprout up along the route of lymphatic drainage** on the arm, with localized lymphadenopathy

6) Treatment: oral potassium iodide (mechanism unclear) or itraconazole

7) Resistance: none

8) Prophylaxis: wear protective gloves/clothing while gardening

2. Invasive Pathogens

   a. *Blastomyces dermatitidis*

     1) Appearance: large round yeast with **thick wall and a broad-based bud** (these are key buzzwords on exams!)

     2) Lab assays: diagnose by biopsy or smear showing the famous broad-based bud

     3) Virulence factors: none significant

     4) Epidemiology: almost identical to *Histoplasma* (see below), transmitted via inhalation of spores from soil, is endemic to the midwestern river valleys and Atlantic states, **key buzz-phrases to look for are travel to the Mississippi, Ohio, or Missouri River Valleys, or East Coast/Atlantic states**

     5) Clinical Diseases:

       a) Pneumonia: causes a subacute pneumonia similar to *Histoplasmosis*

       b) Disseminated disease: similar to *Histoplasmosis* (see below)

     6) Treatment: itraconazole for pneumonia, amphotericin for disseminated disease

     7) Resistance: none

     8) Prophylaxis: none

   b. *Candida spp.*

     1) Appearance: **mucous membrane lesions appear like cottage cheese**, KOH prep of skin lesions show yeast and **pseudohyphae** (germ tubes sprout from yeast but do not form complete hyphae) (see Figure 2)

     2) Lab assays: *C. albicans* species can be identified by the germ tube assay, when placed in serum *C. albicans* will form germ tubes within minutes

     3) Virulence factors: avidly adheres to plastic and forms biofilm on plastic so it cannot be eradicated once it is seeded

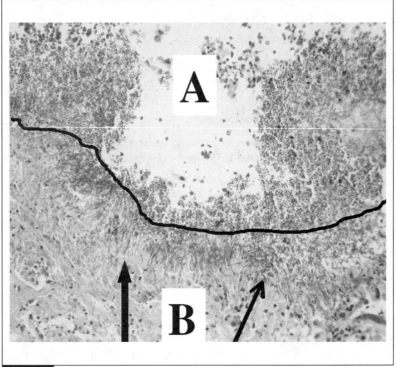

FIGURE 2

Candida *invading tissue. The slide is artificially divided in half with A) showing the typical necrotic tissue left in the wake of the advancing fungus, and B) showing an advancing line of* Candida *hyphae (thick arrow) and pseudohyphae (thin arrow). Pseudohyphae are intermediate stages between yeast and hyphae, and therefore contain a spherical remnant of the yeast form as well as an elongating protrusion which will develop into the hyphal form. On silver staining, all fungi appear black against a light blue-green background.*

4) Epidemiology: normal flora of skin and GI tract, causes thrush in newborns, diabetics, or those with poor T cell-mediated immunity, such as AIDS patients—**intriguingly, it does not cause invasive disease in patients with T cell defects, but it does cause severe, invasive disease in patients with phagocyte defects (usually neutropenics), and even more interestingly it tends not to cause thrush in these patients**

5) Clinical Diseases:

a) Thrush: mucous membrane infection in young, diabetic, or T cell deficient patients

b) UTI: seen in nursing home or hospitalized patients, **usually associated with placement of Foley catheter**

c) Fungemia: **seen in patients with in-dwelling catheters (especially central lines), neutropenic patients, patients who have undergone bowel surgery, patients on long-term parenteral nutrition, or patients receiving broad spectrum antibiotics** (wipes out normal flora, allowing *Candida* to proliferate)—mortality in neutropenic patients is 50% even with first-line therapy

d) Organ seeding: fungemic **patients frequently seed the eye** (always perform funduscopic exam), the liver and spleen causing microabscesses, the kidney, and can also seed the meninges, iv drug abusers can seed heart valves

6) Treatment:

a) Thrush: oral fluconazole or topical nystatin swish and swallow

b) UTI: change or remove the Foley catheter, treat with amphotericin bladder washes or oral fluconazole

c) Fungemia/organ seeding: **remove/change all in-dwelling lines,** in non-neutropenic patients oral fluconazole and iv amphotericin are equivalently efficacious, treat neutropenics with iv amphotericin

7) Resistance: **non-*albicans* species are frequently resistant to azole drugs**

8) Prophylaxis: sterile catheter placement, change lines and Foley catheters regularly, avoid broad-spectrum antibiotics if possible

c. *Coccidioides immitis*

1) Appearance: **giant spherules with thick walls, filled with dozens of smaller endospores, particularly visible on silver stain** (see Figure 3)

2) Lab assays: grows as mold in soil but spherule in tissue, diagnose by biopsy or serology, culturing poses hazards to lab personnel

3) Virulence factors: none significant

4) Epidemiology: transmitted via inhalation of spores which grow in soil in **southwestern US** (central and southern California, especially desert areas, New Mexico, Arizona, Texas), **look for several key**

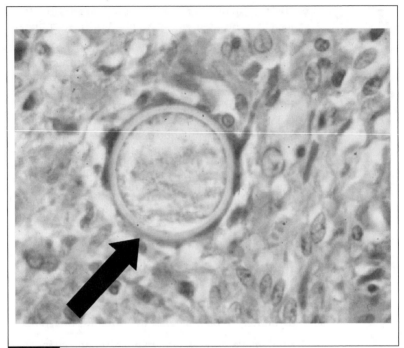

FIGURE 3

A giant Coccidioides spherule seen in tissue. The spherule contains dozens of yeast forms within its tough walls.

buzz-phrases in exam questions: travel to southwestern US desert, archaeological expedition (due to close contact with soil), **time proximity to earthquake** (disruption of soil by shaking often causes outbreaks)

5) Clinical Diseases:

   a) Pneumonia: San Joaquin Valley Fever (named for a valley in Central California): usually occurs in people traveling through the southwestern US (not natives), presents with **TB-like constitutional symptoms,** fevers, weight loss, chronic cough, and also can present with **erythema nodosum** (good prognostic sign), **CXR shows infiltrate with hilar adenopathy**

   b) Disseminated disease: **increased likelihood in African–Americans and Filipinos** (for unclear reasons, but known not to be linked to MHC), as well as in immunocompromised patients, causes

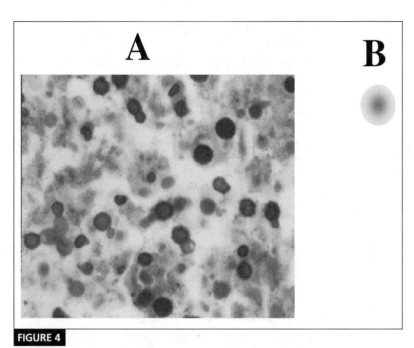

FIGURE 4

A) **Cryptococcus** *yeast in tissues. B) In CSF, India Ink stain reveals yeast surrounded by a thick, clear, polysaccharide capsule. The India Ink does not stain the polysaccharide, leaving the appearance of a "halo" around the yeast.*

disseminated skin lesions, as well as hepatosplenic granulomas, and can disseminate to meninges causing severe meningitis, look for hypercalcemia (a sign of disseminated granulomatous disease)

6) Treatment: fluconazole for pneumonia, fluconazole or amphotericin plus flucytosine for meningitis

7) Resistance: none

8) Prophylaxis: avoid southwestern desert areas

d. *Cryptococcus neoformans*

1) Appearance: oval budding yeast with large capsule (see Figure 4)

2) Lab assays: **India Ink preparation (especially of CSF) reveals small spherical organism surrounded by giant white "halo"** which is the polysaccharide capsule, can also send CSF and serum for CRAG (*Cryptococcal* antigen)

3) Virulence factors: polysaccharide capsule inhibits phagocytosis

4) Epidemiology: transmitted via aerosolization of **pigeon droppings** (or other birds)

5) Clinical Diseases: Meningitis: **usually in AIDS patients but non-AIDS patients do develop the disease if organism burden is high enough** (consider the diagnosis in a case scenario involving a pigeon farmer!), disease disseminates in AIDS patients, causing skin lesions and organ seeding

6) Treatment: amphotericin plus flucytosine intravenously, followed by oral fluconazole suppression

7) Resistance: none

8) Prophylaxis: no primary prophylaxis (except to avoid pigeon guano!), but all patients who develop the disease should receive chronic fluconazole for secondary prophylaxis

e. *Histoplasma capsulatum*

1) Appearance: biopsy shows oval yeast, sometimes found within macrophages (see Figure 5)

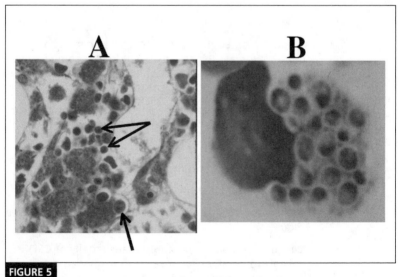

FIGURE 5

A) Appearance of **Histoplasmosa** *yeast (arrows) in a section of lung. B) Appearance of a clump of* **Histoplasma** *in peripheral blood.*

2) Lab assays: **urine *Histoplasma* antigen is highly reliable,** organism grows as mold in soil but spherule in tissue

3) Virulence factors: none significant

4) Epidemiology: transmitted via inhalation of spores which are carried at **high burdens in bat guano and bird droppings,** is endemic to the midwestern river valleys, **key buzz-phrases to look for are exposure to bats, spelunking expedition (people who climb in caves and get exposed to bats), travel to the Mississippi, Ohio, or Missouri River Valleys, or the patient recently cleaned his/her chicken coops**

5) Clinical Diseases:

    a) Pneumonia: causes a subacute pneumonia similar to *Coccidioides* and TB, **CXR shows infiltrates and hilar adenopathy**

    b) Disseminated disease: occurs in immunocompromised, like *Cocci* it causes disseminated skin lesions, as well as hepatosplenic granulomas, and can disseminate to meninges causing severe meningitis, look for hypercalcemia (a sign of disseminated granulomatous disease)

6) Treatment: itraconazole for pneumonia, amphotericin for disseminated disease

7) Resistance: none

8) Prophylaxis: avoid bat guano, be careful when cleaning chicken coops, be wary while on those frequent spelunking expeditions

f. *Pneumocystis carinii* (prior to DNA analysis, was considered a protozoa)

1) Appearance: clumps of cysts best seen on silver staining (see Figure 6)

2) Lab assays: silver stain and culture of bronchoscopic washings are necessary for the diagnosis

3) Virulence factors: none significant

4) Epidemiology: ubiquitous fungus, which almost always **causes diseases in AIDS patients or patients on chronic steroids**

5) Clinical Diseases: Pneumonia (PCP): typically a subacute presentation followed by a sudden decompensation in

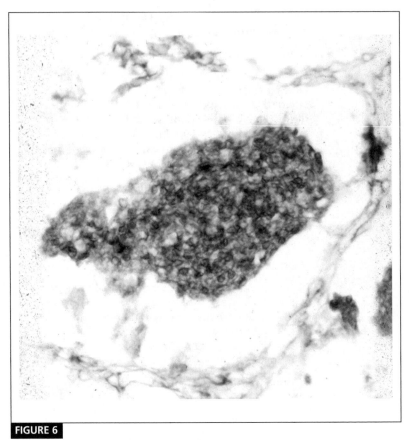

FIGURE 6

Silver stain revealing a large clump of **Pneumocystis** *within an alveola.*

function, **with severe hypoxia and dyspnea out of proportion to unimpressive lung exam, CXR shows "ground glass" haziness in bilateral lower lobes, pleural effusions are distinctly rare and their presence should make one reconsider the diagnosis, patients typically have markedly elevated LDH** which comes down with treatment

6) Treatment: intravenous Bactrim plus prednisone taper

7) Resistance: unusual

8) Prophylaxis: **all AIDS patients with CD4 counts <200 should be on Bactrim prophylaxis**

TABLE 14	Summary of Invasive Yeast	
	APPEARANCE	**EPIDEMIOLOGY**
Candida	Pseudohyphae	Normal flora, risk factors for fungemia: (1) catheters, (2) GI surgery, (3) broad spectrum antibiotics, (4) neutropenia, (5) parenteral nutrition
Cryptococcus	Giant halo in India Ink	Aerosolized pigeon droppings, usually in AIDS
Coccidioides	Giant spherules filled with endospores	Inhaled spores from soil in SW US states, ↑ risk dissemination in African American or Filipinos
Histoplasma	Oval yeast within macrophages	Inhalation of spores in bat or bird guano, endemic to midwestern river valleys
Blastomyces	Thick-walled yeast with broad-based bud	Inhalation of spores from soil, endemic to midwestern river valleys and Atlantic states
Pneumocystis	Silver-stained cysts	Ubiquitous, causes disease in AIDS or other T cell deficiency (e.g., steroid treatment)

B. Molds

1. Cutaneous Pathogens

   a. Dermatophytoses (Microsporum, Trichophyton, Epidermophyton)

   1) Appearance: KOH prep of skin lesions show hyphae

   2) Lab assays: none significant

   3) Virulence factors: none significant

   4) Epidemiology: ubiquitous, spread by direct contact or fomites

   5) Clinical Diseases: Cause the common conditions of athlete's foot (tinea pedis), jock-itch (tinea cruris), and ringworm

   6) Treatment: topical azole cream

   7) Resistance: none

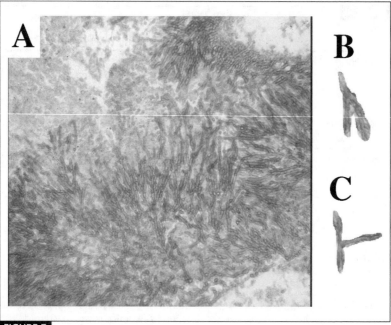

FIGURE 7

A) **Aspergillus** *hyphae invading lung tissue.* **Aspergillus** *causes extensive tissue necrosis, visible in the upper left corner of the image. B) A close-up image of an individual* **Aspergillus** *hyphus, revealing the characteristic 45° angle at which the hyphae branch. C) For comparison, a 90° angle of branching typical of the mold,* **Mucor.**

        8) Prophylaxis: good hygiene

  2. Invasive Pathogens

    a. *Aspergillus fumigatus*

      1) Appearance: **septate hyphae with branching at 45° angles** (see Figure 7)

      2) Lab assays: IgE titers for *Aspergillus* are high in allergic bronchopulmonary Aspergillosis

      3) Virulence factors: none significant

      4) Epidemiology: ubiquitous organism, transmission is airborne via soil or fresh vegetation

      5) Clinical Diseases:

        a) **Fungus ball**: the organism **colonizes cavities formed by prior necrotizing disease, commonly**

from old tuberculosis, and causes hemoptysis, rarely becomes invasive

b) Invasive Pulmonary Aspergillosis: **seen in neutropenic patients or those on chronic steroids,** causing hemoptysis, dyspnea, and even pneumothorax, as disease progresses hypoxia can become severe

c) Allergic Bronchopulmonary Aspergillosis: **a hypersensitivity reaction to fungus** in the large airways, acts very similar to asthma, high titers of IgE specific for the organism are helpful in diagnosis

d) Disseminated disease: **usually in neutropenics,** or patients on chronic steroids, can seed any organ, highly lethal

6) Treatment:

a) Fungus ball: amphotericin B

b) Invasive Pulmonary Aspergillosis: amphotericin B plus surgical resection

c) Allergic Bronchopulmonary Aspergillosis: itraconazole

d) Disseminated disease: amphotericin B and G-CSF to speed bone marrow recovery—disseminated disease has a mortality >50% even with amphotericin

7) Resistance: not intrinsically resistant to amphotericin B *in vitro*, but difficult to treat *in vivo*

8) Prophylaxis: neutropenic precautions = strict hand washing, no fresh fruits or vegetables, no intramuscular injections, etc.

b. Mucormycosis (*Mucor* and *Rhizopus*)

1) Appearance: **nonseptate hyphae with branching at 90° angles** (see Figure 7-C)

TABLE 15	Summary of Invasive Molds	
	APPEARANCE	**EPIDEMIOLOGY**
Aspergillus	Septate hyphae, 45° branches	Neutropenics and chronic steroid
Mucormycosis	Non-septate hyphae, 90° branches	Diabetic ketoacidosis and neutropenics

TABLE 16	Overall Summary of Fungi	
	KEY WORD/PHRASES	**TREATMENT**
Cutaneous Yeast		
Malassezia	• Tinea versicolor • Fluoresces under Woods lamp	Topical azole cream
Sporothrix	• Inoculated via thorn puncture of skin • Spreads up lymphatics of arm	Potassium iodide or itraconazole
Invasive Yeast		
Blastomyces	• Microscope → "thick wall, broad-based bud" • Indigenous to midwestern river valleys and Atlantic states • Very similar clinically to *Histoplasma*	Itraconazole (not fluconazole), amphotericin for disseminated disease
Candida	• Cottage cheese appearance • Risk for mucosal dz = T cell defects (AIDS) • Risks for invasive dz = neutropenia, ICU, multiple catheters, broad-spectrum antibiotics, GI surgery	Fluconazole for non-neutropenics, amphotericin B for neutropenics
Coccidioides	• Indigenous to southwestern US deserts • Exposure to soil (e.g., archaeological expedition or yard work) and time proximity to earthquakes • Mimics TB clinically • Hilar adenopathy and erythema nodosum • Filipinos and African–Americans much higher risk of developing disseminated dz	Fluconazole or amphotericin (for severe disease)
Cryptococcus	• Meningitis in AIDS patients • India Ink test positive in CSF • Pigeon droppings loaded with *Cryptococcus*	Amphotericin, then fluconazole for life
Histoplasma	• Indigenous to midwestern river valleys • Bat and bird guano contain the organism • Exposure to caves (e.g., spelunking) or cleaning of chicken coops • Like *Cocci*, mimics TB	Itraconazole (not fluconazole), amphotericin for disseminated disease

TABLE 16	*Continued*	
	KEY WORD/PHRASES	**TREATMENT**
Pneumocystis	• Silver stain of bronchoscopy makes dx • Almost always in AIDS pts • Insidious dyspnea with abrupt decline in course • CXR shows "ground glass" haziness • Markedly elevated LDH	Bactrim plus prednisone
Cutaneous Molds		
Microsporum, Trichophyton, Epidermo- phyton	• Athlete' s foot • Jock itch • Ringworm	Topical azole cream
Invasive Molds		
Aspergillus	• Septate hyphae with 45° branches • Fungus ball on CXR • Neutropenia almost always present	Amphotericin B
Mucormycosis	• Non-septate hyphae with 90° branches • Ketoacidosis most common risk • Also seen in neutropenics • Starts with subtle headache or visual loss	Surgery plus amphotericin B

2) Lab assays: none

3) Virulence factors: none significant

4) Epidemiology: ubiquitous on decaying vegetation, can be transmitted via inhalation or direct skin contact

5) Clinical Diseases: **rhinocereberal mucormycosis is almost exclusively seen in diabetic patients in ketoacidosis** (the acidity is the key to susceptibility, not just high glucose) or in neutropenic patients, a deadly, invasive disease usually starting in the sinuses which erodes through the skull, into the eyes and brain, typically presents (especially on the boards) with a bad headache or acute vision change in a diabetic in ketoacidosis—**always think of *Mucor* in a diabetic with a headache or vision change**

6) Treatment: surgical resection and amphotericin B, the amphotericin alone only halts the spread to further tissue, but does nothing for already infected tissue

7) Resistance: not intrinsically resistant to amphotericin B *in vitro*, but difficult to treat *in vivo*

8) Prophylaxis: none

IV. PARASITES

A. Protozoa

1. GI/GU

a. *Cryptosporidium*

1) Appearance: cysts are small, **stain pink in stool specimens**

2) Lab assays: stool O&P

3) Virulence factors: none significant

4) Epidemiology: ubiquitous but **typically causes disease in AIDS patients**

5) Clinical Diseases: watery diarrhea, causes severe malabsorption in AIDS patients

6) Treatment: supportive

7) Resistance: none

8) Prophylaxis: boil or filter water, chlorination does not work

b. *Entamoeba histolytica*

1) Appearance: two phases of life-cycle: cyst has four nuclei, trophozoite has one nucleus and is not flagellated **and often contains ingested red blood cells** (see Figure 8)

2) Lab assays: stool O&P should reveal cyst or trophozoite, anti-amoeba antibody titers are diagnostically useful

3) Virulence factors: none significant

4) Epidemiology: fecal-oral transmission

5) Clinical Diseases: amoebic dysentery and amoebic liver abscess

6) Treatment: metronidazole for the bowel infection, and iodoquinol for the liver infection

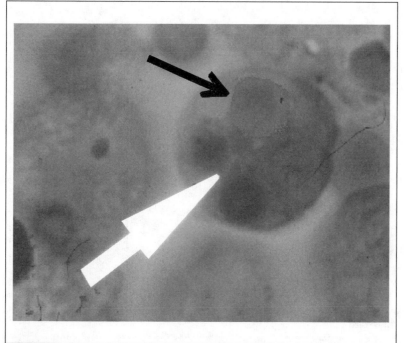

FIGURE 8

Classic **Entameoba** *cyst (light arrow) with an ingested red blood cell (dark arrow).*

7) Resistance: none

8) Prophylaxis: boil or filter water, chlorination has no effect, careful hand-washing and separation of human wastes from crop-fields (don't fertilize crops with human feces)

c. *Giardia lamblia*

1) Appearance: two phases of life-cycle: cyst has four nuclei and has a thicker wall than *Entamoeba*, **trophozoite is oval with two nuclei and has four pairs of flagella** (see Figure 9)

2) Lab assays: stool O&P, string test = patient swallows a string down into the duodenum while the physician holds onto the far end and then pulls the string back up out of the mouth, revealing the trophozoites stuck onto the string

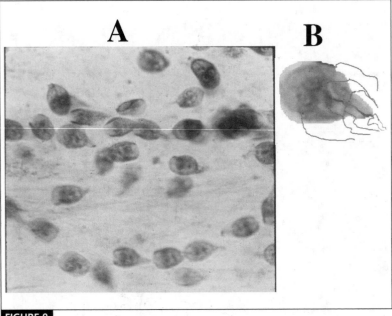

A

B

FIGURE 9

A) Typical appearance of **Giardia** *trophozoites from an intestinal biopsy.*
B) Close-up of an individual trophozoite, revealing the presence of two nuclei and four pairs of flagella.

   3) Virulence factors: none significant

   4) Epidemiology: fecal-oral transmission, often via streams in the wilderness as many animals carry *Giardia* as well, **classic Boards scenario is a hiker who drinks from a stream and gets diarrhea, disease is common in patients with IgA deficiency**

   5) Clinical Diseases: chronic diarrhea, no tissue invasive disease

   6) Treatment: metronidazole

   7) Resistance: none

   8) Prophylaxis: boiling or filtering water, chlorination doesn't work

d. *Trichomonas*

   1) Appearance: there is no cyst stage, **pear-shaped trophozoite, with four flagella, highly motile on wet-mount**

TABLE 17	Summary of GI/GU Protozoa		
ORGANISM	**APPEARANCE**	**DISEASE**	**TREATMENT**
Cryptosporid-ium	Cyst stain pink in stool, nuclei not visible	Watery diarrhea, typically in AIDS	Supportive
Entamoeba	Thin-walled cyst with 4 nuclei, **trophozoite ingests red blood cells and is not flagellated**	Bloody diarrhea, invasive hepatic abscess	Metronidazole and iodoquinol
Giardia	Thick-walled cyst with 4 nuclei, **trophozoite is oval and has 4 pairs of flagella**	Non-bloody diarrhea, often in hikers	Metronidazole
Trichomonas	No cyst, **trophozoite is oval with 4 single flagella**	Vaginitis	Metronidazole (treat both sex partners)

2) Lab assays: wet mount

3) Virulence factors: none significant

4) Epidemiology: sexually transmitted, resides in the vagina or, rarely in male GU tract, can be spread by asymptomatic carriers

5) Clinical Diseases: vaginitis with **green, frothy discharge, can cause urethritis in men, watch out for Boards questions where both the male and female sex partners have GU symptoms, or questions in which the female is diagnosed with *Trichomonas* and treated appropriately but comes back shortly with a new infection— both sex partners must be treated simultaneously to eradicate the disease**

6) Treatment: metronidazole, treat both sex partners

7) Resistance: none

8) Prophylaxis: condoms

2. Invasive protozoa

a. *Babesia*

1) Appearance: intracellular ring forms within red cells similar to malaria

2) Lab assays: blood smear, serology

3) Virulence factors: none significant

4) Epidemiology: transmitted via tick bite, **typically occurs in the New England area, specifically along the coast**

5) Clinical Diseases: high fevers, shaking chills, myalgias, abdominal pain, nausea/vomiting, followed by **severe hemolytic anemia particularly dangerous in splenectomized patients**

6) Treatment: clindamycin plus quinine

7) Resistance: none

8) Prophylaxis: avoid tick bites

b. *Leishmania spp.*

1) Appearance: amastigotes are small intracellular organisms seen within macrophages

2) Lab assays: blood smear or tissue biopsy reveal organisms within macrophages, serologies often positive

3) Virulence factors: none significant

4) Epidemiology: transmitted via sandfly bite, visceral disease seen in Asia and Africa, cutaneous disease seen in Central and South America as well as Asia and Africa, mucocutaneous disease seen only in Central and South America

5) Clinical Diseases:

a) **Kala-azar = visceral leishmaniasis: caused by** *L. donovani*, organism is concentrated in the reticuloendothelial system (liver, spleen, lymph nodes, bone marrow), causing **massive hepatosplenomegaly, pancytopenia,** hemorrhage, and susceptibility to secondary infections, patients also get hyperpigmented skin

b) **Cutaneous leishmaniasis: caused by** *L. tropica* (Old World disease in Asia and Africa) **and** *L. mexicana* (New World disease in Central/South America), disease starts with **erythematous papule at site of sandfly bite,** can either heal spontaneously or progress to large, granulomatous ulcerations which often is secondarily infected by bacteria

c) **Mucocutaneous leishmaniasis: caused by** *L. braziliensis,* **also starts as papule at site of sandfly bite, but can disseminate to multiple mucosal spots,** creating granulomatous erosions of nose and mouth

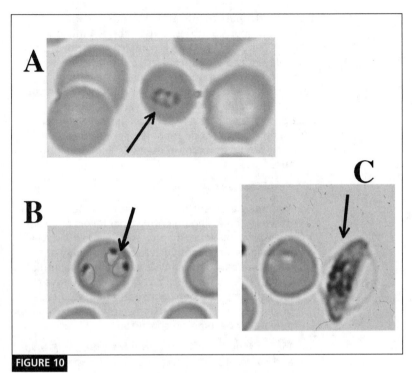

FIGURE 10

A) and B) show typical "signet ring" schizonts of malaria in red blood cells. C) shows the classic "crescent" shaped gametocyte of **P. falciprum** *found in peripheral blood.*

6) Treatment: sodium stibogluconate

7) Resistance: unusual

8) Prophylaxis: long-sleeve shirts, long pants, insect repellents, pesticides to kill sandflies

c. *Plasmodium* (**malaria**): *falciparum, vivax, ovale, malariae*

1) Appearance: schizonts appear like **"signet rings"** in red blood cells, while the gametocyte of *P. falciprum* appears like a large crescent attached to a thin ring (see Figure 10)

2) Lab assays: thin and thick smear of whole blood to detect trophozoites

3) Virulence factors: none significant

4) Epidemiology: **transmitted by bite of *Anopheles* mosquito, infects several hundred million people**

worldwide, particularly affects Africa and all Mediterranean countries, **causes about 1 million deaths per year,** life cycle is complicated: sporozoites inoculated into blood from mosquito bite, seed the liver and transform into merozoites, leave the liver and infect red blood cells, transform into trophozoite which multiplies and then transforms back into merozoites and bursts the red cell, infects new red cells and then the cycle repeats—**note that** *P. ovale* **and** *P. vivax* **can lie dormant in the liver, allowing long-term relapse**

5) Clinical Diseases:

   a) General characteristics: all four species cause a cluster of symptoms including **paroxysmal fevers and shaking rigors, myalgias, diaphoresis, severe headache, arthralgias, and signs such as splenomegaly and hepatomegaly, red cell lysis causes anemia, initially the fever is continuous, but after several days the red cell bursts become synchronized in** *P. vivax, ovale,* **and** *malariae* **infections, note that** *falciparum* **may never become synchronized**

   b) **Tertian fever:** synchronous red cell bursts in *P. vivax* **and** *ovale* cause tertian fevers (**q48 hr** = tertian because it occurs on the 3rd day, it is not q3 days), **relapse is common in tertian fever because** *vivax* **and** *ovale* **have a latent phase in the liver**

   c) **Quartan fever:** synchronous red cell bursts in *P. malariae* causes quartan fevers (**q72 hr** because it occurs on the 4th day, it is not q4 days)

   d) *P. falciparum* **can cause continuous or irregular fevers without patterns, the organism burden in** *P. falciparum* **infections is much higher, and the red cells become sticky and can clog capillaries and cause DIC, leading to strokes and renal failure, CNS disease in a malaria patient is almost always due to** *P. falciparum,* **and carries a very high mortality**

6) Treatment:

   a) Tertian fever: if *P. vivax* or *ovale* **proven or suspected, treat with chloroquine (for merozoites in blood) plus primaquine (for latent organisms in liver)**—beware pts with G6PDH deficiency, in whom quinine-derivatives cause dangerous hemolytic anemia

TABLE 18	Summary of *Plasmodium spp.*			
ORGANISM	**FEVER TIMING**	**CNS DZ**	**LATENT?**	**TREATMENT***
Falciparum	Irregular or q48 hr	Yes	No	CQ
Vivax/ovale	q48 hr	No	Yes	CQ + PQ
Malariae	q72 hr	No	No	CQ
*Assumes not resistant, CQ = chloroquine, PQ = primaquine.				

b) *P. falciparum* and Quartan fever: if *P. falciparum* or *malariae* proven or suspected, treat with chloroquine alone (primaquine not needed since there is no latent liver phase)—beware pts with G6PDH deficiency

7) Resistance: an increasingly severe problem, resistance endemic in South America, Africa, SE Asia, and parts of Middle East with few proven alternatives to quinine-derivatives, quinine plus doxycycline may cover some resistant organisms, other regimens are so unusual they are not likely testable on the USMLE

8) Prophylaxis:

a) Mosquito netting and DEET insect repellent are keys to avoid inoculation—it is much more effective to prevent bites than to prevent infection due to increasing drug resistance

b) Chemoprophylaxis depends on if travel is to area with resistant organism

i) Non-resistant area (Central America north of the Panama Canal, some parts of the Middle East and some parts of the Caribbean): chloroquine for several weeks before the trip, during the trip, and for several weeks after the trip

ii) Resistant area: mefloquine or doxycycline for before, during the trip, and after the trip

d. *Toxoplasma gondii*

1) Appearance: biopsy of infected tissue reveals crescent-shaped organisms

2) Lab assays: IgM serologies to detect acute infection

3) Virulence factors: none significant

4) Epidemiology: **transmitted via the feces of kittens (older cats less likely)**, or via ingestion of poorly cooked meat containing cysts, can also be transmitted vertically if the mother is newly infected during pregnancy

5) Clinical Diseases:

   a) Immunocompetent people either get asymptomatically exposed or develop **mild heterophile negative mononucleosis**

   b) AIDS patients: **clinical disease primarily seen in HIV patients,** immunosuppression allows dissemination of the organism classically causing severe **encephalitis with multiple ring-enhancing lesions in the brain**

   c) Congenital: causes multi-organ disease and can lead to spontaneous abortion or severe congenital retardation

6) Treatment: pyrimethamine plus sulfamethoxazole plus folinic acid (folinic acid is used to prevent folate deficiency caused by the drugs—**note that folate cannot be used because folate is upstream of the drug-induced block in the biosynthetic pathway, folinic acid is used because it is downstream of the block**) or intravenous Bactrim

7) Resistance: none, but alternative therapies are required in sulfa-allergic patients

8) Prophylaxis: AIDS patients and pregnant women should avoid kittens and should not clean kitty litter, cook meats thoroughly, **AIDS patients with CD4 count <200 per μl should be on Bactrim prophylaxis**

e. *Trypanosoma*

   1) Appearance: large, crescentic trypomastigotes seen in blood, smaller, circular amastigotes seen in tissues

   2) Lab assays: biopsy and serologies

   3) Virulence factors: **antigenic shift**—the organism can shift its surface antigens as antibody responses develop, keeping it one step ahead of the immune response

   4) Epidemiology: *T. cruzi* **transmitted via reduviid bug,** endemic to Central and South America, which bites the patient and then passes organism through the broken skin by defecating in the bite wound, *T. gambiense* **and**

TABLE 19	Summary of Invasive Protozoa		
	TRANSMISSION	**EPIDEMIOLOGY**	**TISSUE TROPISM**
Babesia	Tick bite	• Coastal New England	Red blood cells
Leishmania	Sandfly bite	• Mucocutaneous dz in Central/South America • Cutaneous dz in Central/South America & Asia/Africa • Visceral dz in Asia/Africa	Macrophages
Plasmodium	*Anopheles* mosquito	Africa, Middle East, Caribbean, Central/South America, SE Asia	RBCs (liver for *P. vivax/ovale*)
Toxoplasma	Cat feces or cysts in undercooked meat	Ubiquitous	Brain
Trypanosoma	• Reduviid bug (*cruzi*) • Tsetse fly (other *spp*)	• Central/South America (*cruzi*) • Africa (other *spp*)	Heart (*cruzi*), CNS (other *spp*)

T. rhodesiense **transmitted by the tsetse fly, endemic to Africa**

5) Clinical Diseases:

    a) Chagas disease: caused by *T. cruzi*, **reduviid bug often bites the face near the eyes, so look for Romana's sign, a swollen/puffy cheek near the eye,** acutely the organism causes lymphoreticular disease with fever, lymphadenopathy, and hepatosplenomegaly, chronic persistence of the organism leads to amastigote invasion of the heart and colon, **causing heart block and myocarditis/dilated cardiomyopathy as well as megacolon, and achalsia**

    b) African Sleeping Sickness: caused by *T. gambiense* and *T. rhodesiense*, presents with an ulcer at the site of the fly bite, **can lead to either an acute, severe encephalitis with rapid decline in CNS function leading to coma, or a chronic course over several years**

6) Treatment:

　　a) Chagas disease: if caught during acute infection, nifurtimox effective, there is no antimicrobial therapy for chronic disease; however, **pacemakers are crucial if heart block develops**

　　b) African Sleeping Sickness: **suramin effective prior to onset of CNS disease** but it doesn't cross the blood brain barrier well, so it is useless once CNS disease sets in

7) Resistance: unusual

8) Prophylaxis: insect netting, insect repellent

B. Metazoa (Multicellular Animals)

1. Tapeworms (cestodes)

　a. *Diphyllobothrium latum*

　　1) Appearance: **longest tapeworm**, up to 30 feet

　　2) Lab assays: stool O&P

　　3) Virulence factors: none significant

　　4) Epidemiology: **acquired by consuming raw, freshwater fish**

　　5) Clinical Diseases: weight loss, diarrhea, **vitamin B12 deficiency**

　　6) Treatment: praziquantel

　　7) Resistance: none

　　8) Prophylaxis: cook fish

　b. *Echinococcus*

　　1) Appearance: small tapeworm

　　2) Lab assays: stool O&P

　　3) Virulence factors: none significant

　　4) Epidemiology: fecal oral transmission from **dog feces, with sheep an important intermediate host—thus shepherds are commonly patients**

　　5) Clinical Diseases: hydatid cysts in any organ of the body, if cysts rupture can cause fatal anaphylaxis

　　6) Treatment: albendazole and careful surgical excystation

7) Resistance: none

8) Prophylaxis: good hygiene

c. *Hymenolepis nana*

1) Appearance: small tapeworm (up to 5 cm long)

2) Lab assays: stool O&P

3) Virulence factors: none significant

4) Epidemiology: fecal oral transmission, with humans as major host

5) Clinical Diseases: typically asymptomatic

6) Treatment: praziquantel

7) Resistance: none

8) Prophylaxis: good hygiene

d. *Taenia saginata* (beef tapeworm)

1) Appearance: tapeworm can be several meters long

2) Lab assays: stool O&P

3) Virulence factors: none significant

4) Epidemiology: **ingestion of undercooked beef**, transmitted to cattle via fecal-oral route

5) Clinical Diseases: typically asymptomatic, although some patients might suffer discomfort (and embarrassment!) due to the **occasional protrusion of the tapeworm tail from the anus**

6) Treatment: praziquantel

7) Resistance: none

8) Prophylaxis: good hygiene

e. *Taenia solium* (pork tapeworm)

1) Appearance: tapeworm can be several meters long

2) Lab assays: stool O&P

3) Virulence factors: none significant

4) Epidemiology: **can be transmitted either by ingestion of larva in undercooked pork causing tapeworm infection of gut, or by ingestion of eggs in food due to fecal contamination,** eggs mature into larva in gut and burrow into tissues, causing cysticercosis

TABLE 20	**Summary of Tapeworms (cestodes)**	
	TRANSMISSION	**CLINICAL Dz**
Diphylloboth-rium	Raw fish	Weight loss, diarrhea, B12 deficiency
Echinococcus	Dog feces or ingestion of infected sheep meat	Often asymptomatic or mass lesions in any organ causes symptoms
Hymenolepis	Human feces	Asymptomatic
Taenia saginata	Undercooked beef	Typically asymptomatic, worm may protrude from anus
Taenia solium	Undercooked pork or human feces	Asymptomatic tapeworm infection, or ingestion of eggs in feces causes cysticercosis, which presents with seizures and chemical meningitis from ruptured cysts in the brain

5) Clinical Diseases:

   a) Tapeworm infection: like *T. saginata*, often asymptomatic

   b) Cysticercosis: space-occupying lesions occur in tissues, often in brain, and death of the larva induces inflammatory response which can cause seizures and chemical meningitis—**new onset seizures in an immigrant from Latin America is neurocysticercosis until proven otherwise**

6) Treatment: praziquantel, steroids and anti-seizure medications often needed in neurocysticercosis

7) Resistance: none

8) Prophylaxis: good hygiene

2. Flukes (trematodes)

  a. *Clonorchis sinensis* (**Asian liver fluke**)

   1) Appearance: not remarkable

   2) Lab assays: stool O&P

   3) Virulence factors: none significant

   4) Epidemiology: **transmitted by ingestion of raw freshwater fish, endemic to Asia**

     5) Clinical Diseases: may be asymptomatic, however, the flukes lodge in the liver and can cause **hepatitis and biliary obstruction** ultimately leading to cirrhosis or hepatocellular carcinoma

     6) Treatment: praziquantel

     7) Resistance: none

     8) Prophylaxis: cook fish

b. *Paragonimus westermani* **(Asian lung fluke)**

     1) Appearance: not remarkable

     2) Lab assays: stool O&P

     3) Virulence factors: none significant

     4) Epidemiology: transmitted by **ingestion of raw crab-meat, endemic to Asia**, organism penetrates intestinal wall, migrates through the diaphragm to the lung and can thus be transmitted either by feces or sputum

     5) Clinical Diseases: chronic cough, hemoptysis and dyspnea

     6) Treatment: praziquantel

     7) Resistance: none

     8) Prophylaxis: cook crab meat

c. *Schistosoma japonicum, mansoni*, and *haematobium*

     1) Appearance: ova are ovoid with sharp protuberance called a spine at one end, *S. haematobium* ova have a big spine at the very terminus of the egg, *S. mansoni* ovum have big spine off to the side (about 2 o' clock if the terminus is 12 noon), while *S. japonicum* have a less prominent spine (see Figure 11)

     2) Lab assays: stool O&P

     3) Virulence factors: none significant

     4) Epidemiology:

        a) infection occurs by direct **penetration of human skin by free-swimming larva, life-cycle requires freshwater environment with snails** (which are intermediate hosts)

        b) *S. mansoni* occurs in tropical areas around the world, including Africa, the Middle East, and South America, but **does not occur in Asia**

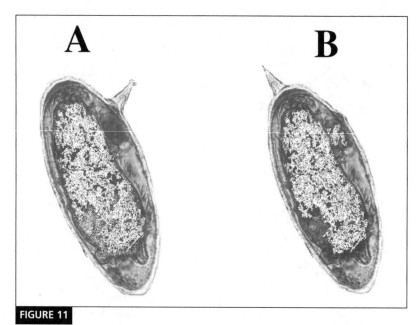

A) The classic appearance of **Schistosoma mansoni,** *with a terminal spine at approximately 2 o' clock. B) In contrast, the spine of* **Schistosoma haematobium** *is at the very terminus (12 o' clock).*

    c) *S. japonicum* **occurs in Asia**

    d) *S. haematobium* occurs in Africa and the Middle East

5) Clinical Diseases:

    a) *S. japonicum & mansoni*: acute infection **causes pruritis and erythematous eruption at the site of skin penetration,** after several weeks fevers and lymphadenopathy begin, tissue penetration causes **marked eosinophilia, adult schistosomes reside in the liver venules and their eggs cause granulomatous reaction in the liver, leading to portal hypertension and hepatosplenomegaly, can induce cirrhosis** leading to all the usual sequelae

    b) *S. hematobium*: **adult worms reside in the bladder venous plexus,** and their eggs cause granulomas and fibrosis in the bladder, leading to **hematuria, can also induce transitional cell carcinoma of the bladder**

6) Treatment: praziquantel

TABLE 21	Summary of Flukes (trematodes)		
	TRANSMISSION	LOCATION	CLINICAL Dz
Clonorchis	Raw freshwater fish	Asia	Hepatitis, biliary obstruction
Paragonimus	Raw crab meat	Asia	Chronic cough, hemoptysis
Schistosoma haematobium	Skin penetration by freshwater larvae	Africa, Middle East	Hematuria, transitional bladder CA
Schistosoma japonicum	Skin penetration by freshwater larvae	Asia	Granulomatous hepatitis, cirrhosis, portal hypertension
Schistosoma mansoni	Skin penetration by freshwater larvae	Africa, Middle East, South America	Granulomatous hepatitis, cirrhosis, portal hypertension

7) Resistance: starting to be seen for *S. mansoni*

8) Prophylaxis: avoid swimming in waters with host snails

3. Intestinal Roundworms (nematodes)

a. *Ascaris lumbricoides*

1) Appearance: large roundworms, can be a foot long, and can form mass-like conglomerations in the intestines (see Figure 12)

2) Lab assays: stool O&P

3) Virulence factors: none significant

4) Epidemiology: fecal-oral transmission of eggs, after ingestion, eggs hatch in the intestine, the larva penetrate the intestinal wall and enter the bloodstream, then the larva escape into the lungs, penetrate the alveoli and are coughed up the trachea so that they are swallowed back down into the intestine where the mature into adults and pass more eggs—**this is the most common parasitic infection in the world, with up to 1 billion people infected**

5) Clinical Diseases: although infection can be asymptomatic, **eosinophilic pneumonia** occurs during larval migration into the alveoli, malnutrition can occur due to adult worms scavenging nutrients in the gut, and

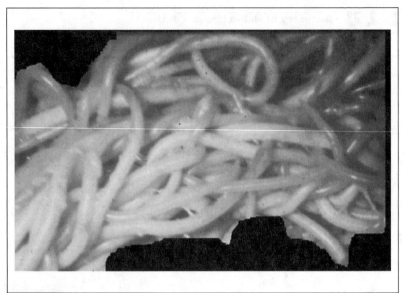

Appearance of a mass of **Ascaris** *worms.*

                  bowel obstruction can occur due to luminal occlusion by large numbers of the large adult worms

      6) Treatment: albendazole or mebendazole, pyrantel pamoate as 2nd line

      7) Resistance: none

      8) Prophylaxis: good hygiene

   b. *Enterobius vermicularis* (pinworm)

      1) Appearance: small white worms, 1 cm or less

      2) Lab assays: scotch tape test = place scotch tape over anus and examine on a slide, the tape picks up the eggs which are visible under the microscope, worms can be directly visualized by stool O&P (but eggs are not present in stool)

      3) Virulence factors: none significant

      4) Epidemiology: **most common helminthic infection in the US**, transmission is fecal-oral, **at night the female worm migrates out the anus and lays eggs in the peri-anal area**

5) Clinical Diseases: **perianal pruritis**

6) Treatment: albendazole or mebendazole, pyrantel pamoate as 2nd line

7) Resistance: none

8) Prophylaxis: good hygiene

c. Hookworm (*Ancylostoma duodenale* and *Necator americanus*)

1) Appearance: long, thin worms, *Necator* has cutting plates to grab hold of the intestinal wall while *Ancylostoma* uses teeth

2) Lab assays: Stool O&P

3) Virulence factors: none significant

4) Epidemiology: ***Ancylostoma duodenale* is found in most of the underdeveloped world (Old World hookworm), while *Necator americanus* (New World hookworm) is found in the southeastern US, infection occurs via direct penetration of skin in contact with moist soil containing larvae,** like *Ascaris* the larvae migrate via blood to the lungs where they are coughed up and swallowed, allowing mature adults to develop in the intestines and to pass eggs in the stool

5) Clinical Diseases: a pruritic, **erythematous dermatitis occurs at the site in the skin where the larvae penetrate, and eosinophilic pneumonia occurs** during transmigration of the larvae through the alveoli, some time after infection iron deficient anemia develops (**hookworm is the #1 cause of iron deficiency anemia in the world**), with all the usual anemia symptoms (e.g., weakness, fatigue, etc.), eosinophilia is typical

6) Treatment: albendazole or mebendazole, pyrantel pamoate as 2nd line

7) Resistance: none

8) Prophylaxis: good sanitation, avoid direct skin contact with contaminated soil (e.g., don't walk barefoot through the soil)

d. *Strongyloides stercoralis*

1) Appearance: small round worms (see Figure 13)

2) Lab assays: stool O&P

3) Virulence factors: none significant

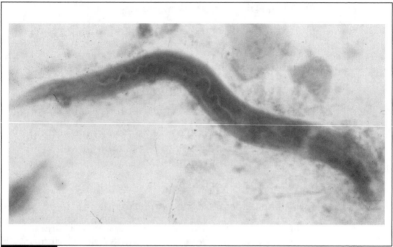

FIGURE 13

Appearance of **Strongyloides** *in the sputum of an infected patient.*

4) Epidemiology: endemic throughout the tropical world, and also in the southeastern US, direct contact of skin with **soil contaminated by feces allows larval penetration into the host**, the larva migrates via blood to the lung where they are coughed up and swallowed, allowing adult maturation in the intestines, the adult worms lay eggs which either are defecated out to start the next cycle, or mature into larva within the infected host, allowing another round of infection within the same host in a process called autoinfection, **autoinfection can lead to overwhelming infection in immunocompromised patients**

5) Clinical Diseases: **Cutaneous Larva Migrans = severe local contact dermatitis occurs at the site of skin penetration**, pts can be asymptomatic, but some develop diarrhea, eosinophilic pneumonia, or sepsis from bacterial translocation across a damaged gut wall, **peripheral eosinophilia is prominent**

6) Treatment: ivermectin or albendazole

7) Resistance: none

8) Prophylaxis: good sanitation, avoid bare skin contact with contaminated soil (e.g., don't walk barefoot through the soil)

TABLE 22	Summary of Intestinal Roundworms (nematodes)	
	TRANSMISSION	**CLINICAL Dz**
Ascaris	Fecal oral	Eosinophilic pneumonia, bowel obstruction
Enterobius	Fecal oral	Perianal pruritis in children
Ancylostoma	Skin penetration by larvae in moist soil	Pruritic, erythematous dermatitis at site of penetration, iron deficient anemia and eosinophilia, occurs in Europe and Asia
Necator	Skin penetration by larvae in moist soil	Pruritic, erythematous dermatitis at site of penetration, iron deficient anemia and eosinophilia, occurs in the SE USA
Strongyloides	Skin penetration by larvae in moist soil	Local contact dermatitis at site of skin penetration, diarrhea, eosinophilic pneumonia, sepsis
Trichuris	Fecal oral	Invasive diarrhea, rectal prolapse
Trichinella	Undercooked pork or game (bear or deer)	Diarrhea, severe myositis, headache, extreme eosinophilia

    e. *Trichuris trichiura* (whipworm)

       1) Appearance: long thin worm, with a thread-like tail extending twice the length of the worm

       2) Lab assays: stool O&P

       3) Virulence factors: none significant

       4) Epidemiology: fecal-oral transmission of eggs, eggs mature into adults in intestine, which then lay more eggs, there is no tissue phase

       5) Clinical Diseases: often asymptomatic, but may cause invasive diarrhea, does NOT typically cause iron-deficient anemia, **in patients with heavy worm burden rectal prolapse can occur**

       6) Treatment: albendazole or mebendazole

       7) Resistance: none

       8) Prophylaxis: good sanitation and good hygiene

    f. *Trichinella spiralis*

    1) Appearance: larvae are oval with ring-like centers, found in tissue, particularly muscle

    2) Lab assays: **muscle biopsy, note stool O&P not helpful, look for marked eosinophilia**

    3) Virulence factors: none significant

    4) Epidemiology: typically transmitted via **ingestion of undercooked pig, bear, or deer meat** containing larvae, larvae mature in the intestine, and lay eggs which penetrate into the bloodstream, seeding striated muscle throughout the body

    5) Clinical Diseases: **Trichinosis:** an initial diarrhea is followed within 2 weeks by **severe myositis, headache with diffuse muscle aches, high fever, and extreme eosinophilia (up to 90% of peripheral white blood cells),** can also cause CNS and cardiac damage

    6) Treatment: albendazole or mebendazole with or without corticosteroids

    7) Resistance: none

    8) Prophylaxis: cook meats thoroughly

4. Tissue Roundworms (nematodes)

  a. *Dracunculus medinensis*

    1) Appearance: coiled worm up to a foot or more long can be seen burrowed beneath the skin, skin typically blisters and then ulcerates over the worm

    2) Lab assays: none

    3) Virulence factors: none significant

    4) Epidemiology: transmission is via **ingestion of fresh-water crustaceans containing larvae,** larvae mature in the intestine and the adult migrates to skin, the disease is on the decline in Africa due to WHO efforts to eradicate

    5) Clinical Diseases: pruritic and painful welts overlying the subcutaneous worm, with ulceration over the worm's head

    6) Treatment: surgical withdrawal of the worm

    7) Resistance: none significant

    8) Prophylaxis: boil or filter suspect drinking water, avoid ingestion

b. *Loa loa*

1) Appearance: can be seen as small (centimeter) subconjunctival worm burrowing across the eye or skin

2) Lab assays: thick and thin smear to identify parasites in the blood

3) Virulence factors: none significant

4) Epidemiology: endemic to Africa, transmitted by the bite of the deer fly

5) Clinical Diseases: **dermatitis or conjunctivitis caused by hypersensitivity to migrating worm in skin or eye**

6) Treatment: diethylcarbamazine, surgical excision may be required for conjunctival infections

7) Resistance: none

8) Prophylaxis: eradication of deer fly vector

c. *Oncocerca volvulus*

1) Appearance: worm less than a millimeter long

2) Lab assays: skin biopsy revealing the parasite

3) Virulence factors: none significant

4) Epidemiology: endemic to Africa, **particularly riverbeds, transmitted by bite of blackfly,** the organisms do not travel through blood, instead migrate subcutaneously

5) Clinical Diseases: **causes "river blindness"** (that's right, the people go blind from worm migration into the eyes, hence the name)

6) Treatment: ivermectin plus corticosteroids for patients with eye infection

7) Resistance: none

8) Prophylaxis: eradicate blackfly vector, ivermectin can be taken prophylactically

d. *Toxocara canis*

1) Appearance: not significant

2) Lab assays: tissue biopsy

3) Virulence factors: none significant

4) Epidemiology: transmitted via **dog feces contaminating soil** and foodstuffs, eggs hatch into larvae in

TABLE 23	Summary of Invasive Roundworms (nematodes)	
	TRANSMISSION	CLINICAL Dz
Dracunculus	Freshwater crustaceans	Welts overlying the subcutaneous worm
Loa	Deerfly bite	Hypersensitivity to migrating worm
Oncocerca	Blackfly bite	Blindness
Toxocara	Dog feces	Visceral larva migrans = diffuse granulomas, retinitis, eosinophilia, headache, myalgias
Wuchereria and *Brugia*	Mosquito bite	Elephantiasis

the intestine, the larvae then disseminate to multiple tissues

5) Clinical Diseases: **"Visceral Larva Migrans" = diffuse granulomatous reactions causing fevers, myalgias, headache, CNS disease and retinal disease**, with a **prominent eosinophilia**, typically presents in children playing in soil with dogs

6) Treatment: treat symptoms with corticosteroids and antihistamines, treatment of worms with diethylcarbamazine is controversial

7) Resistance: none

8) Prophylaxis: good sanitation and hygiene

e. *Wuchereria bancrofti* **and** *Brugia malayi*

1) Appearance: worm less than a millimeter long

2) Lab assays: thick blood smears with blood drawn at night

3) Virulence factors: none significant

4) Epidemiology: **Wuchereria is endemic to Africa while Brugia is endemic to Asia** (particularly Malaysia hence the species name *malayi*), **both transmitted by mosquito bites**, organisms mature in lymph nodes and then circulate in the blood, particularly at night

5) Clinical Diseases: **elephantiasis**, obstruction of lymphatics leads to severe lymphedema

TABLE 24	**Overall Summary of Parasites**	
	KEY WORD/PHRASES	**TREATMENT**
GI/GU Protozoa		
Cryptosporid-ium	• Diarrhea in AIDS patient	Supportive
Entamoeba	• Amoebic dysentery • Amoebic liver abscess	Metronidazole plus iodoquinol
Giardia	• Chronic non-bloody diarrhea in a hiker/camper	Metronidazole
Trichomonas	• Vaginitis with green, frothy discharge • Frequent recurrences because sexual partner needs treatment as well	Metronidazole
Invasive Protozoa		
Leishmania	• Sandfly bite in Asia, Africa, Latin America • Cutaneous ulcer • Lymphadenopathy, hepatosplenomegaly	Sodium stibogluconate
Plasmodium	• Mosquito bite in Africa, Mediterranean, Latin America • Shaking rigors, severe headache, myalgias • Cyclical fevers	Chloroquine ± primaquine
Toxoplasma	• Exposure to kitten feces or poorly cooked meat • Typically in AIDS pts with ring-enhancing brain lesions	Pyrimethamine + sulfametho-xazole + folinic acid
Trypanosoma	• Reduviid bug bite in Latin America • Tsetse fly bite in Africa • Romana' s sign = swelling near eye where bite occurred • Heart block in a young person • Megacolon	Nifurtimox or suramin acutely, nothing works for chronic dz
Tapeworms (cestodes)		
Diphyllobot-hrium	• Raw fish consumption • B12 deficiency	Praziquantel
Echinococcus	• Shepherds, exposure to dogs and sheep • Large cysts seen in liver or lung	Albendazole and surgery
Hymenolepis	• Dog feces	Praziquantel
Taenia saginata	• Undercooked beef • Tapeworm protrusion from anus	Praziquantel

TABLE 24	*Continued*	
	KEY WORD/PHRASES	**TREATMENT**
Taenia solium	• Undercooked pork or fecal-oral • Seizures and encephalitis in a Hispanic person	Praziquantel ± seizure medicine
Flukes (trematodes)		
Clonorchis	• Asian liver fluke • Raw freshwater fish	Praziquantel
Paragonimus	• Asian lung fluke • Raw crab meat	Praziquantel
Schistosoma	• Swimming in freshwater with snails nearby • Portal hypertension • Hematuria, bladder cancer	Praziquantel
Intestinal Roundworms (nematodes)		
Ascaris	• Eosinophilic pneumonia • Bowel obstruction • Iron deficiency	Albendazole
Enterobius	• Kid with itchy anus • Small white worms seen near anus • Eggs picked up from anus with scotch-tape	Albendazole
Ancylostoma	• Dermatitis at site of contact with moist soil • Iron deficiency anemia	Albendazole
Necator	• Dermatitis at site of contact with moist soil • Iron deficiency anemia • Southeastern US, poor areas	Albendazole
Strongyloides	• Local contact dermatitis (cutaneous larva migrans) at site of contact with moist soil • Eosinophilic pneumonia, auto infection	Ivermectin or albendazole
Trichuris	• Rectal prolapse	Albendazole
Trichinella	• Undercooked pig, bear, or deer meat • Severe myalgias with extreme eosinophilia	Albendazole

TABLE 24	*Continued*	
	KEY WORD/PHRASES	**TREATMENT**
Invasive Roundworms (nematodes)		
Dracunculus	• Long worm seen coiled beneath skin	Worm extraction
Loa	• Small worm seen underneath conjunctiva	Diethylcarbamazine
Oncocerca	• Blackfly bite • River blindness in Africa	Ivermectin
Toxocara	• Visceral Larva Migrans • Retinal disease • Prominent eosinophilia	Steroids, antihistamines, ? diethylcarbamazine
Wuchereria (Brugia)	• Elephantiasis	Ivermectin

6) Treatment: ivermectin effective against larvae but not adult worms

7) Resistance: none

8) Prophylaxis: prevention of mosquito bites

V. VIRUSES

A. DNA Viruses

1. Naked DNA Viruses (unencapsulated)

   a. Adenovirus

   1) Genome: linear, double stranded DNA

   2) Lab assays: none significant

   3) Virulence factors: none significant

   4) Epidemiology: ubiquitous, airborne, fecal-oral, and fomite transmission, **outbreaks common in communal living situations,** e.g., military barracks

   5) Clinical Diseases: **mucosal infections,** including URIs, mild gastroenteritis, conjunctivitis, **classic illness is**

"**pharyngoconjunctival fever,**" a combination conjunctivitis with pharyngitis

6) Treatment: supportive

7) Resistance: not applicable

8) Prophylaxis: good hygiene, vaccine in use by the military

b. Papovaviruses

1) Human Papillomavirus (HPV)

a) Genome: circular, double stranded DNA

b) Lab assays: none significant

c) Virulence factors: HPV E6 and E7 proteins are carcinogenic, inactivating p53 and the retinoblastoma (Rb) proto-oncogenes, respectively

d) Epidemiology: ubiquitous, transmission by direct contact, especially through damaged skin

e) Clinical Diseases:

   i) HPV serotypes 1–4 cause common skin warts

   ii) HPV serotypes 6–11 cause genital warts

   iii) **HPV serotypes 16, 18, 31, 33, 35 cause cervical cancer, and are sexually transmitted**

f) Treatment: freezing for skin warts, caustic application (e.g., podophyllin or salicylic acid) for genital warts, surgical excision with or without adjunctive radio- and chemotherapy for cervical cancer

g) Resistance: not applicable

h) Prophylaxis: good hygiene and safe sex

2) Polyomaviruses: JC virus and BK virus

a) Genome: circular, double stranded DNA

b) Lab assays: none significant

c) Virulence factors: none significant

d) Epidemiology: affect immunocompromised, **JC seen in AIDS patients and BK seen in renal transplant patients**

e) Clinical Diseases:

   i) **JC Polyomavirus causes Progressive Multifocal Leukoencephalopathy in AIDS patients,** a

TABLE 25	Summary of Naked DNA Viruses	
VIRUS	**TRANSMISSION**	**DISEASE**
Adenovirus	Airborne, fecal-oral, & fomite	Conjunctivitis, pharyngitis, URI, gastroenteritis, classic dz is **pharyngoconjunctival fever**
HPV	Skin contact	Warts, cervical cancer
JC Polyomavirus	Unknown	Progressive Multifocal Leukoencephalopathy in AIDS
BK polyomavirus	Unknown	Nephritis, renal graft rejection in transplant patients
Parvovirus B19	Contact	• 5th dz ("slapped cheek" viral exanthem) in kids • Aplastic anemia in chronic hemolysis patients • Hydrops fetalis in placental transmission to fetus

          relentlessly progressive encephalopathy which is almost invariably fatal

    ii) **BK Polyomavirus causes severe nephritis in transplanted kidneys**

  f) Treatment: none

  g) Resistance: not applicable

  h) Prophylaxis: none

c. Parvovirus B19

  1) Genome: single stranded DNA

  2) Lab assays: serologies and PCR assay

  3) Virulence factors: none significant

  4) Epidemiology: ubiquitous, transmitted by contact, pregnant women should be isolated from infected patients due to the risk of transmission to the fetus

  5) Clinical Diseases:

    a) **Fifth Disease**: also known as erythema infectiosum or "slapped-cheek" disease, a mild viral exanthem seen in children causing **bright red erythema of the cheeks and lacy exanthem on the arms and trunk**, self-limiting

b) **Aplastic anemia: Parvovirus B19 infxn of chronic hemolysis pts** (e.g., Sickle Cell) can trigger aplastic crisis, **as the virus selectively infects stem cell precursors of RBCs,** particularly when stem cells are replicating quickly (↑ replication during hemolysis as the body tries to repopulate RBCs)

c) Hydrops fetalis: transplacental transmission can be lethal to the fetus

d) Immune deposition arthritis develops in adults following URI

6) Treatment: supportive

7) Resistance: not applicable

8) Prophylaxis: good hygiene

2. Encapsulated DNA Viruses

a. Hepadnavirus Family

1) Hepatitis B Virus (HBV)

a) Genome: circular, incompletely double stranded DNA

b) Lab assays:

i) **Hepatitis B Surface Antigen** (HBsAg) **levels in serum indicate active infection**

ii) **Hepatitis B Surface Antibody** (HBsAb) **levels in serum indicate immunity to the virus,** during the development of immunity as the HBsAb titers rise, the surface antigen titers fall to undetectable

iii) **Hepatitis B Core Antibody** (HBcAb) **levels in serum also indicate active infection, but they rise before surface antibody rises and are therefore positive in the window period when the surface antigen has fallen to undetectable but the surface antibody isn't yet detectable**

iv) **The Hepatitis B E Antigen is expressed during viral replication, and is a marker for high risk of transmission due to active viral shedding**

v) Viral DNA levels in serum allow detection of active infection

c) Virulence factors: interesting life cycle, in which the virus transcribes its genome into mRNA and then uses reverse transcriptase (of HIV fame) to generate a new DNA genome from the mRNA

d) Epidemiology: transmitted by body fluid contamination, most often via sexual transmission or IV drug abuse, but also via tattoo needles and blood transfusions (extremely rare now), but note that although rare in the US, **the #1 mode of transmission in the world is vertical, occuring in Asia where millions of infants are born with the virus**

e) Clinical Diseases:

  i) Acute viral hepatitis with the usual fever, myalgias, nausea, vomiting, jaundice, transaminitis, the virus is cleared by 90% of patients

  ii) Chronic hepatitis: **10% of people who contract the disease as adults fail to clear the virus, but 90% of children who acquire the virus vertically fail to clear the virus,** leading to either an asymptomatic carrier state or chronic active hepatitis with nausea, vomiting, persistent transaminitis, immune-complex glomerulonephritis

  iii) Cirrhosis: occurs in patients with chronic active hepatitis

  iv) Hepatocellular carcinoma: develops in some people with chronic active hepatitis—**the risk of carcinoma is particularly high in children who acquire the disease vertically, and hepatocellular carcinoma is the most common malignancy in the world because of the incredibly high prevalence in Asia where vertical transmission is common**

f) Treatment: lamivudine (an inhibitor of reverse transcriptase) or interferon-α

g) Resistance: often develops

h) Prophylaxis: the Hepatitis B vaccine is a recombinant surface antigen with a >90% efficacy rate, recommended for health care workers, patients with underlying liver disease, drug abusers or anyone else at high risk for acquiring the virus—some recommend everyone be vaccinated

b. The Herpes Virus Family

  1) Cytomegalovirus (Human Herpes Virus 5)

   a) Genome: linear, double-stranded DNA

   b) Lab assays: direct fluorescent antibody (DFA), serologies, but >75% adults have positive titers

   c) Virulence factors: none significant

   d) Epidemiology: transmitted by body fluid contamination, often via saliva or sexual transmission, also vertically and via organ transplants

   e) Clinical Diseases:

      i) Vertical transmission causes multiorgan disease, can be fatal to the fetus or infant, and is a common cause of mental retardation

      ii) Adult infection is often asymptomatic

      iii) **Viral syndrome indistinguishable from mononucleosis only heterophile antibody test is negative**

      iv) **Disseminated disease occurs in immunocompromised patients, can cause a granulomatous hepatitis, severe pneumonitis,** kidney disease, induce kidney graft rejection in transplant patients, and in AIDS patients causes diarrhea and vision threatening chorioretinitis

   f) Treatment: ganciclovir

   g) Resistance: none

   h) Prophylaxis: good hygiene to avoid exposure

2) Epstein-Barr Virus (EBV)(Human Herpes Virus 4)

   a) Genome: linear, double-stranded DNA

   b) Lab assays: **heterophile antibody (Monospot test)**

   c) Virulence factors: binds to CD21 on B cells to initiate viral uptake

   d) Epidemiology: transmission is via saliva, >90% adults have been exposed

   e) Clinical Diseases:

      i) **Mononucleosis,** with fever, malaise, somnolence, and extensive lymphadenopathy with hepatosplenomegaly

      ii) EBV has been associated with Burkitt's lymphoma and non-Hodgkin's lymphoma, although causality has not been rigorously proven

f) Treatment: none

g) Resistance: not applicable

h) Prophylaxis: none

3) Herpes Simplex Virus-1 (HSV-1) (Human Herpes Virus 1)

   a) Genome: linear, double-stranded DNA

   b) Lab assays: Serology, DFA, Tzanck prep = scraping of base of an ulcer which on Wright–Giemsa stain reveals a clump of multinucleated giant cells, PCR of CSF

   c) Virulence factors: none significant

   d) Epidemiology: transmitted via saliva

   e) Clinical Diseases: typically causes cold sores, oral ulcers, conjunctivitis, and temporal lobe meningoencephalitis **(note these are all infections of cranium)**

   f) Treatment: acyclovir

   g) Resistance: latent virus is resistant, acyclovir only works during active outbreaks

   h) Prophylaxis: good hygiene

4) Herpes Simplex Virus-2 (HSV-2) (Human Herpes Virus 2)

   a) Genome: linear, double-stranded DNA

   b) Lab assays: Serology, DFA, Tzanck prep = scraping of base of an ulcer which on Wright–Giemsa stain reveals a clump of multinucleated giant cells, PCR of CSF

   c) Virulence factors: none significant

   d) Epidemiology: **transmitted via sexual contact**

   e) Clinical Diseases: typically causes **vesicles that erode into ulcers on the genitals,** can also cause oropharyngeal ulcers after oral sex, neonatal herpes can occur after transit of the infant through an infected vaginal canal, can also cause meningitis

   f) Treatment: acyclovir

   g) Resistance: latent virus is resistant, acyclovir only works during active outbreaks

   h) Prophylaxis: safe sex

5) Human Herpes Virus 6 (HHV 6) & 7 (HHV 7)

      a) Genome: linear, double-stranded DNA

      b) Lab assays: none

      c) Epidemiology: probably transmitted via saliva

      d) Clinical Diseases: **Roseola infantum**, a childhood exanthem in which the child feels fine despite a high fever which lasts for up to 5 days, after the fever breaks a maculopapular rash erupts over the trunk and limbs and then resolves within about 24 hr

      e) Treatment: none

      f) Resistance: not applicable

      g) Prophylaxis: none

6) Human Herpes Virus 8 (HHV 8)

      a) Genome: linear, double-stranded DNA

      b) Lab assays: none

      c) Virulence factors: none significant

      d) Epidemiology: transmitted via sexual contact, particularly anoreceptive intercourse

      e) Clinical Diseases: **HHV 8 strongly associated with Kaposi's sarcoma in AIDS patients but causal link not quite proven yet**, can also cause a much milder growth of endothelium seen in immunocompetent adults from the Mediterranean region

      f) Treatment: chemoradiotherapy for Kaposi's Sarcoma, none for the virus

      g) Resistance: not applicable

      h) Prophylaxis: safe sex

7) Varicella-Zoster Virus (VZV) (Human Herpes Virus 3)

      a) Genome: linear, double-stranded DNA

      b) Lab assays: can use serologies and Tzanck prep, but diagnosis is almost always clinical

      c) Virulence factors: **becomes latent in dorsal root ganglia**, allowing recrudescence after many years

      d) Epidemiology: transmitted is airborne

      e) Clinical Diseases:

          i) **Chicken pox**, a highly infectious childhood illness marked by classic, **pruritic, vesicular rash,** appearing like a "dew-drop on a rose" with a central clearing on an erythematous macule, immunity to first infection is usually lifelong so repeat episodes of chicken pox are rare

    ii) **Zoster, a reactivation disease usually seen in the immunocompromised or elderly, presents with a highly characteristic dermatomal vesicular rash and severe neuropathic pain along a dermatomal distribution, note that the pain can precede the rash by several days, so always think of Zoster if there is dermatomal pain even if no rash is apparent**

  f) Treatment: acyclovir

  g) Resistance: none

  h) Prophylaxis: vaccine is now available, recommended for all children and unexposed adults

c. Poxviruses

  1) Molluscum contagiosum

    a) Genome: linear, double-stranded DNA

    b) Lab assays: biopsy

    c) Virulence factors: none significant

    d) Epidemiology: transmitted via direct contact with skin or fomites

    e) Clinical Disease: causes a classic papular rash, with papules that have pearly surface with **umbilicated center, can cause diffuse papules in AIDS patients**

    f) Treatment: liquid nitrogen freezing of papules

    g) Resistance: none

    h) Prophylaxis: good hygiene

  2) Smallpox (Variola)

    a) Genome: linear, double-stranded DNA

    b) Lab assays: none

    c) Virulence factors: none significant

    d) Epidemiology: transmitted via direct contact with skin or fomites and by respiratory droplets, natural infection has been eradicated from the world, but several laboratories around the world have frozen stocks

TABLE 26	Summary of Encapsulated DNA Viruses			
VIRUS	**TRANSMIS- SION**	**DISEASE**	**TREAT- MENT**	**VACCINE?**
Hepadnavirus				
HBV	Body fluids, vertical	Acute & chronic hepatitis, cirrhosis, hepatocellular carcinoma	Lamivu- dine or IFN-α	Yes
Herpes Virus Family				
Cytomega- lovirus	Body fluids, organ transplant, vertical	• Vertical transmission → mental retardation and death • Adults →asymptomatic or heterophile-negative mono • AIDS →diarrhea, hepatitis chorioretinitis, pneumonitis • Transplant pts → nephritis, hepatitis, pneumonitis	Gancicl-ovir	None
EBV	Saliva	Mononucleosis, ? lymphomas	Suppor-tive	None
HSV-1	Saliva	Cold sores, conjunctivitis, meningoencephalitis	Acyclovir	None
HSV-2	Sexual	Genital vesicles and ulcers	Acyclovir	None
HHV 6 & 7	Saliva	Roseola infantum	None	None
HHV 8	Sexual	Kaposi' s sarcoma*	None	None
Varicella-Zoster	Airborne	Chicken pox, zoster	Acyclovir	Yes
Poxvirus				
Molluscum contagios-um	Skin contact	Skin papules with umbilicated centers	Mecha-nical removal	None
Smallpox	Airborne or contact	Eradicated from world, caused papular rash and pneumonitis	None	Yes

*Strong link found between HHV 8 and Kaposi' s sarcoma, but causality not yet proven.

      e) Clinical Disease: caused diffuse papular-pustular rash and disseminated disease with pneumonitis

      f) Treatment: none

      g) Resistance: none

      h) Prophylaxis: vaccine in widespread use

B. RNA Viruses

1. Naked RNA Viruses (unencapsulated)

   a. Caliciviruses

      1) Hepatitis E Virus

         a) Genome: single-stranded RNA

         b) Lab assays: none significant

         c) Virulence factors: none significant

         d) Epidemiology: fecal-oral transmission

         e) Clinical Diseases: acute viral hepatitis much like hepatitis A virus; **however, note that hepatitis E virus causes high mortality in pregnant women**

         f) Treatment: supportive

         g) Resistance: not applicable

         h) Prophylaxis: none

      2) Norwalk Virus

         a) Genome: single-stranded RNA

         b) Lab assays: none significant

         c) Virulence factors: none significant

         d) Epidemiology: fecal-oral transmission, **often via undercooked shellfish**

         e) Clinical Diseases: acute viral gastroenteritis, typically self-limited

         f) Treatment: supportive

         g) Resistance: not applicable

         h) Prophylaxis: none

   b. Picornaviruses

      1) Enteroviruses (so-called because they are transmitted via the gastrointestinal, or "entero-," mucosa)

a) Coxsackievirus

   i)   Genome: single-stranded RNA

   ii) Lab assays: none significant

   iii) Virulence factors: none significant

   iv) Epidemiology: fecal-oral and airborne transmission

   v) Clinical Diseases:

      a)) Aseptic meningitis: **one of the most common causes**

      b)) Herpangina: pharyngitis with vesicles in posterior oropharynx

      c)) Hand–Foot–Mouth dz: vesicles on hands and feet, with ulcers in oropharynx

      d)) Myocarditis: a **dilated cardiomyopathy**, which can spontaneously resolve or can result in progressive congestive heart failure, causing death

      e)) Serositis: pericarditis and pleuritis

      f)) URI: mild flu-like illness

   vi) Treatment: supportive

   vii) Resistance: not applicable

   viii) Prophylaxis: none

b) Echovirus

   i)   Genome: single-stranded RNA

   ii) Lab assays: none significant

   iii) Virulence factors: none significant

   iv) Epidemiology: fecal-oral transmission

   v) Clinical Diseases: **one of the most common causes of aseptic meningitis**, also URI

   vi) Treatment: supportive

   vii) Resistance: not applicable

   viii) Prophylaxis: none

c) Hepatitis A Virus (HAV)

   i)   Genome: single-stranded RNA

ii) Lab assays: serology

iii) Virulence factors: none significant

iv) Epidemiology: fecal-oral transmission

v) Clinical Diseases: often asymptomatic, but in some pts causes acute viral hepatitis with fevers, abdominal pain, jaundice, dark urine, myalgias, transaminitis, very rare cause of fulminant hepatic failure

vi) Treatment: supportive

vii) Resistance: not applicable

viii) Prophylaxis: an effective vaccine is available

d) Poliovirus

i) Genome: single-stranded RNA

ii) Lab assays: none significant

iii) Virulence factors: **replicates in anterior horn motor neurons, causing neuronal death and paralysis**

iv) Epidemiology: **fecal-oral transmission,** natural infection eradicated in the developed world

v) Clinical Diseases: **the vast majority of infections are totally asymptomatic, some people develop a flu-like viral syndrome which is self-limited, others develop meningitis, and some develop paralytic poliomyelitis,** note there is also a post-polio syndrome causing progressive myopathy and neuropathic pain, decades after initial clinical infection

vi) Treatment: supportive

vii) Resistance: not applicable

viii) Prophylaxis:

a)) Salk vaccine: an injectable killed poliovirus

b)) Sabin vaccine: an oral attenuated virus

c)) **Although Sabin used to be preferred, in the developed world there are now more cases of polio due to reversion to wild type of the attenuated Sabin vaccine than due to natural polio infections, therefore the Salk vaccine is typically administered for at least the**

VIRUS	TRANSMIS- SION	DISEASE	VACCINE?
TABLE 27 Summary of Naked RNA Viruses			
Calicivirus (single-stranded RNA)			
Hepatitis E Virus	Fecal-oral	Acute viral hepatitis, **note high mortality in pregnant women**	None
Norwalk Virus	Fecal-oral	Acute viral gastroenteritis, often after consumption of undercooked shellfish	None
Picornavirus (single-stranded RNA)			
Enteroviruses			
Coxsackie- virus	Fecal-oral, airborne	• Aseptic meningitis • Herpangina/Hand–Foot–Mouth disease • Myocarditis • Serositis • URI	None
Echovirus	Fecal-oral	Aseptic meningitis and URI	None
Hepatitis A Virus	Fecal-oral	Hepatitis	Yes
Poliovirus	Fecal-oral	Ranges from asymptomatic to URI to meningitis to paralytic polio, also post-polio degenerative disease	Yes (Sabin and Salk)
Rhinoviruses (single-stranded RNA)			
Rhinovirus	Airborne	Common cold	None
Reovirus Family (double-stranded RNA)			
Rotavirus	Fecal-oral	Diarrhea	None

> first two doses while the Sabin can be used for boosters
>
> d)) **The Sabin vaccine should never be used for immunocompromised patients**

2) Rhinovirus ("rhino-" = nose)

   a) Genome: single-stranded RNA

   b) Lab assays: none significant

   c) Virulence factors: binds to the ICAM-1 receptor on respiratory epithelium to mediate its uptake into human host, >100 serotypes makes vaccine development problematic

d) Epidemiology: airborne transmission and fomites

e) Clinical Diseases: **common cold**

f) Treatment: supportive

g) Resistance: not applicable

h) Prophylaxis: good hygiene

c. Reoviruses

1) Rotavirus

a) Genome: double-stranded RNA

b) Lab assays: none significant

c) Virulence factors: none significant

d) Epidemiology: fecal-oral transmission

e) Clinical Diseases: viral gastroenteritis, **Rotavirus is the most common cause of diarrhea worldwide,** usually affecting children ≤2 years old

f) Treatment: supportive

g) Resistance: not applicable

h) Prophylaxis: good hygiene

2. Encapsulated RNA Viruses

a. Positive RNA polarity (genomic RNA directly codes for protein)

1) Coronaviruses

a) Coronavirus, multiple serotypes

i) Genome: single-stranded RNA

ii) Lab assays: none

iii) Virulence factors: none significant

iv) Epidemiology: airborne

v) Clinical Diseases: **common cold, 2nd most common cause behind Rhinoviruses**

vi) Treatment: none

vii) Resistance: not applicable

viii) Prophylaxis: none

2) Flaviviruses

  a) Dengue Virus

    i)   Genome: single-stranded RNA

    ii) Lab assays: none significant

    iii) Virulence factors: none significant

    iv) Epidemiology: an arbovirus (transmitted by insect), transmitted by *Aedes* mosquito found in tropical areas, typical US cases from tourists to the Caribbean

    v) Clinical Diseases:

      a)) **Breakbone fever: severe flu-like syndrome, with unusually striking myalgias and arthralgias (pt feels like bones are breaking!)**, rash is also common, although pt feels awful, breakbone fever is rarely fatal

      b)) **Dengue Hemorrhagic Fever:** starts like breakbone fever, but then diffuse mucosal hemorrhaging begins, typically from GI tract and skin, and shock ensues, frequently fatal

    vi) Treatment: supportive

    vii) Resistance: not applicable

    viii) Prophylaxis: insect repellent, avoid mosquitoes

  b) Hepatitis C Virus (HCV)

    i)   Genome: single-stranded RNA

    ii) Lab assays: serology, viral DNA levels in serum to detect active infection

    iii) Virulence factors: none significant

    iv) Epidemiology: transmitted via blood, by IVDA, needle-sticks, or blood transfusions, the possibility of sexual transmission is somewhat controversial

    v) Clinical Diseases: acute viral hepatitis, **up to 90% of people become chronically infected,** many of whom will end up with cirrhosis or hepatocellular carcinoma

    vi) Treatment: ribavirin and interferon-α, **a combination of the two has been proven to work better than either alone**

vii) Resistance: some serotypes are commonly resistant

viii) Prophylaxis: avoid blood exposures, don't use drugs

c) Yellow Fever Virus

   i)   Genome: single-stranded RNA

   ii)   Lab assays: none

   iii) Virulence factors: none significant

   iv) Epidemiology: an arbovirus (transmitted by insect), transmitted by the *Aedes* mosquito found in tropical Africa and South America

   v)   Clinical Diseases: **a severe viral syndrome causing hepatitis and which can progress to hemorrhagic fever**, often fatal

   vi) Treatment: none

   vii) Resistance: not applicable

   viii) Prophylaxis: avoid mosquitoes, a live-attenuated vaccine is available and is recommended for travelers to endemic areas

3) Retroviruses

a) Human Immunodeficiency Virus (HIV)

   i)   Genome: single-stranded RNA, two copies per virus (diploid)

   ii)   Lab assays:

       a)) **ELISA to screen for anti-HIV antibody,** 99% sensitive, 95% specific

       b)) **Western blot to confirm positive ELISA,** 95% sensitive, 99% specific

       c)) p24 antigen assay to directly detect virus in a patient who has not yet had time to develop antibody to the virus (can take up to 6 months)

       d)) Viral RNA can be directly quantified by PCR or by branched-DNA assays

       e)) CD4 T cell count to determine stage of disease (<200/µl = advanced AIDS)

   iii) Virulence factors:

a)) **gp120** on the viral envelope **binds to CD4** and a 2nd co-receptor on T cells and other cells, the 2nd co-receptor is any of a number of chemokine receptors such as CCR5 and CXCR4

b)) All retroviruses have *gag* genes coding for structural proteins, *pol* genes coding for reverse transcriptase, and *env* genes coding for viral envelop proteins

c)) **HIV *gag* codes for a precursor to the p24 antigen** used clinically to detect infection during acute seroconversion syndrome, before patient's antibody response is positive—note that **protease inhibitors act against a viral protease which cleaves a large precursor viral protein into p24 and several other proteins**

d)) **HIV *pol* protein codes for reverse transcriptase**

e)) **HIV *env* protein codes for gp160,** which is spliced by a host protease into gp120 and gp41—note that protease inhibitors do NOT work against the protease which cleaves gp160, this is a host cell protease

f)) The mechanism of HIV-mediated destruction of CD4+ T cells is unclear; however, it probably relates to some combination of induction of CD8+ T-cell responses against HIV-infected CD4 cells, suppression of thymic selection of new T-cells, direct CD4+ T-cell lysis, and exhaustion of bone marrow lymphocyte stem cells

iv) Epidemiology:

a)) Worldwide heterosexual and vertical transmission is the most common mode, in the US homosexual transmission is still the most common but is decreasing in incidence while heterosexual transmission and IVDA transmission are increasing

b)) Africa has the most cases in the world now, but the most rapid spread is occuring in Southeast Asia and central Europe c)) In the developed world, the death rate from AIDS has plummeted in the last 5 years, but it is not decreased in the underdeveloped world

d)) HIV has two major serotypes, HIV-1 and HIV-2, and dozens of clades which are subtypes of HIV-1

e)) HIV-2 is virtually exclusively found in Western Africa, whereas HIV-1 is the dominant serotype found throughout the rest of the world

f)) **Without therapy, 95% of HIV-infected patients die from AIDS, but up to 5% of patients are Long Term Non-progressors who never become ill from HIV** due to a variety of factors including remarkably potent host response to the virus, infection by defective virus, and host mutations in viral co-receptors such as CCR5 and CXCR4

v) Clinical Disease: acute infection causes a mono-like seroconversion syndrome with rash and sometimes meningitis, then an asymptomatic phase sets in for several years while CD4+ T-cells are steadily destroyed, followed by onset of AIDS in which CD4 counts plummet, making the person susceptible to both common infections like *Streptococcus pneumonia* pneumonia, opportunistic infections, and malignancies caused by viruses and immune dysregulation (e.g., Kaposi's Sarcoma and high grade B-cell lymphomas)

vi) Treatment:

a)) Highly Active Antiretroviral Therapy (HAART): **all patients with HIV should be receiving three or more drugs at a time**, including some combination of a viral nucleoside analogue, a protease inhibitor, and/or a non-nucleoside reverse transcriptase inhibitor

b)) **The overall success of HAART is about 60% at reducing the viral load below the limit of detectability, and the principle cause of HAART-failure is non-compliance with the** complicated regimens that have many unpleasant side effects

c)) **All HIV⊕ patients with CD4 counts <200/μl should be on Bactrim prophylaxis for** *Pneumocystis carinii* **pneumonia (PCP) and** *Toxoplasma*

d)) **All HIV⊕ patients with CD4 counts <50/μl should be on azithromycin prophylaxis for** *Mycobacterium avium intracellulare* **infection**

vii) Resistance: **invariable if treated with less than three drugs, and will occur despite any regimen if compliance is poor**

viii) Prophylaxis: avoid unprotected sex, sharing needles, and needle-sticks, avoid mucosal splashes with body secretions

b) Human T-cell Leukemia Virus (HTLV)

   i) Genome: single-stranded RNA

   ii) Lab assays: serology

   iii) Virulence factors: ability to integrate into host DNA causing cellular transformation

   iv) Epidemiology: transmitted via blood-products and unsafe sex, **HTLV is most prevalent in Japan and in the Caribbean,** there are two dominant serotypes, HTLV-1 and HTLV-2

   v) Clinical Diseases:

      a)) Human T cell leukemia and cutaneous T cell lymphomas

      b)) **Tropical spastic paraparesis: a condition of degeneration of spinal motor neurons leading to hyperspasticity and paresthesias of** the lower extremities accompanied by incontinence of urine and neuropathic pain

   vi) Treatment: none

   vii) Resistance: not applicable

   viii) Prophylaxis: avoid exposure to blood-products and unsafe sex

4) Togaviruses

   a) Encephalitis Viruses

    i)   Genome: single-stranded RNA

    ii)   Lab assays: serology, CSF culture

    iii) Virulence factors: none significant

    iv) Epidemiology:

        a)) All are arboviruses ("arthropod-borne") transmitted by mosquitoes, with wild birds acting as normal hosts

        b)) Eastern Equine Encephalitis Virus is the most severe, with a case fatality rate approaching 50%

        c)) Western Equine Encephalitis Virus causes less severe infections

        d)) St. Louis Encephalitis Virus has a case fatality rate between Eastern and Western Equine Viruses

    v)   Clinical Diseases: encephalitis which is often fatal in the young or elderly

    vi) Treatment: supportive

    vii) Resistance: not applicable

    viii) Prophylaxis: avoid mosquitoes

  b) Rubella

    i)   Genome: single-stranded RNA

    ii)   Lab assays: serology, CSF culture

    iii) Virulence factors: none significant

    iv) Epidemiology: airborne transmission, can be trans-placentally transmitted

    v)   Clinical Diseases: trans-placental transmission causes congenital cardiac, neurological, and ocular malformations, **childhood infection causes the German measles, with a fever and maculopapular rash which is self-limiting**

    vi) Treatment: supportive

    vii) Resistance: not applicable

    viii) Prophylaxis: live-attenuated vaccine

b. Negative RNA polarity (genomic RNA must be transcribed into a complementary strand which codes for protein, thus these viruses require their own RNA polymerase)

1) Arenaviruses

   a) Lymphocytic Choriomeningitis (LCM) Virus

      i)   Genome: single-stranded RNA

      ii) Lab assays: none significant

      iii) Virulence factors: none significant

      iv) Epidemiology: exact mode of transmission unclear, but **exposure to house mice or other rodents is a requisite**

      v) Clinical Diseases: a flu-like illness with rash and leukopenia which can within days progress to **aseptic meningitis of unusual severity, and which may be fatal**

      vi) Treatment: supportive

      vii) Resistance: not applicable

      viii) Prophylaxis: avoid rodents

   b) Lassa Fever Virus

      i)   Genome: single-stranded RNA

      ii) Lab assays: none significant

      iii) Virulence factors: none significant

      iv) Epidemiology: exact mode of transmission unclear, but exposure to rodents and direct human contact are involved, most cases occur in West Africa

      v) Clinical Diseases: a flu-like illness that can progress to cause disseminated disease, including cranial nerve deficits, hepatitis, and **microcapillary leak leading to hemorrhagic fever and shock**

      vi) Treatment: supportive

      vii) Resistance: not applicable

      viii) Prophylaxis: avoid rodents

2) Bunyaviruses

   a) California Encephalitis Virus

      i)   Genome: single-stranded RNA

      ii) Lab assays: serology

      iii) Virulence factors: none significant

      iv) Epidemiology: an arbovirus, spread by mosquitoes, actually occurs over much of North America

      v) Clinical Diseases: encephalitis, typically in children and teens

      vi) Treatment: supportive

      vii) Resistance: not applicable

      viii) Prophylaxis: avoid mosquitoes

   b) Hantavirus

      i) Genome: single-stranded RNA

      ii) Lab assays: serology

      iii) Virulence factors: none significant

      iv) Epidemiology: **spread by inhalation of dust particles from house mice feces, cases typically reported in desert areas like Nevada, New Mexico, and Arizona**, exposure typically in rural area the summer after a wet spring when the rodent population increases

      v) Clinical Diseases: **a flu-like illness which can rapidly progress in hours to Acute Respiratory Distress Syndrome (ARDS),** and has a fatality rate of >50%

      vi) Treatment: supportive

      vii) Resistance: not applicable

      viii) Prophylaxis: rodent population control

3) Deltavirus

   a) Hepatitis D Virus (HDV)

      i) Genome: single-stranded RNA

      ii) Lab assays: serology

      iii) Virulence factors: none significant

      iv) Epidemiology: transmitted by body fluids, typically IVDA or sex, the virus is defective and **cannot replicate unless Hepatitis B Virus co-infects the same cell,** in which case HDV can use proteins made by HBV to replicate

      v) Clinical Diseases: **simultaneous infection of HBV and HDV leads to an acute hepatitis** somewhat more severe than HBV infection alone; **however, if a person is already infected with HBV and then gets HDV on top, it can cause a very severe hepatitis which can progress to fulminant hepatic failure**

      vi) Treatment: supportive

      vii) Resistance: not applicable

      viii) Prophylaxis: safe sex, don't use drugs, immunization with HBV vaccine

4) Filoviruses

    a) Ebola & Marburg Viruses

      i) Genome: single-stranded RNA

      ii) Lab assays: serology

      iii) Virulence factors: none significant

      iv) Epidemiology: mode of transmission not entirely clear, seems to be direct contact with infected body fluids from human to human, although respiratory transmission may also occur, the virus has some unknown reservoir in the tropical jungles of Africa, and how it is transmitted from this reservoir to humans is not known

      v) Clinical Diseases: **flu-like illness progresses to hemorrhagic fever,** with microangiopathic capillary destruction and bleeding from every orifice, causing circulatory collapse, a frighteningly **high mortality rate approaching 80–90%**

      vi) Treatment: supportive, immune serum from convalescing patients has been transfused to newly infected patients during outbreaks, but efficacy is not established

      vii) Resistance: not applicable

      viii) Prophylaxis: none

5) Orthomyxoviruses

    a) Influenza

      i) Genome: segmented, single-stranded RNA (unlike Paramyxoviruses which have single piece of RNA, Orthomyxoviruses have their RNA chopped up into segments, Influenza has eight of these segments)

ii) Lab assays: culture, rapid influenza ELISA

iii) Virulence factors:

a)) **Hemagglutinin binds to host cells to mediate uptake** and **neuraminidase cleaves the virus free of the membrane** to allow the virus to enter the cytoplasm of the infected cell

b)) **Antigenic drift** is the **progressive, steady mutation of the hemagglutinin and neuraminidase** which allows the virus to come back each year with a slightly different structure so that prior acquired immunity is less effective

c)) **Antigenic shift is due to sudden genetic recombination of hemagglutinin and neuraminidase with other influenza types, causing instant generation of brand new viral strains**

d)) Antigenic shift totally negates the effect of prior immunity, since a wholly new virus is created which no immune system has ever seen, and this is responsible for periodic pandemics which can kill millions across the globe every few decades

e)) There are also three serotypes of Influenza, called Types A, B, and C, with **A being the most common etiologic agent of human disease**

iv) Epidemiology: airborne transmission, new viral strains are typically generated in Asia and then spread west across the globe

v) Clinical Diseases: Influenza is different than the common cold, with **high fever, striking myalgias** (particularly of the long muscles in the back and in the hamstrings), cough and headache, **but vomiting, diarrhea, and rhinorrhea are typically NOT present**, in elderly patients secondary **bacterial infections can set in during the resolution phase of Influenza infections, causing a biphasic presentation** of severe illness, followed by recovery, followed by sudden decompensation with cough newly productive of purulent sputum

  vi) Treatment:

    a)) Neuraminidase inhibitors (oseltamivir and zanamivir) are effective at decreasing the severity of Influenza A and B infections and shortening their duration by a day or two if started within 48 hr of onset of symptoms

    b)) Amantadine and rimantadine are only active against Influenza A and also must be started within 48 hr of symptoms to be effective

  vii) Resistance: none described

  viii) Prophylaxis:

    a)) Killed vaccine contains mixture of Influenza A & B and **is reformulated every year based on serotypes causing disease each year, but protection lasts <1 yr so yearly revaccination required**

    b)) Vaccine recommended for: pts > 50 yr old (new rec as of 2000), pts with co-morbid dz (e.g., heart, lung, liver, kidney dz, diabetes, cancer), close contacts of such people, **and health care workers**

    c)) A live-attenuated inhaled vaccine awaits FDA approval

    d)) Amantadine can prevent Influenza A (but not B), useful for elderly contacts of pts with the flu

6) Paramyxoviruses

  a) Measles Virus

    i)   Genome: single-stranded RNA

    ii) Lab assays: serology

    iii) Virulence factors: none significant

    iv) Epidemiology: airborne transmission

    v)   Clinical Diseases: **childhood exanthem with a classic 3 C's of cough, coryza, and conjunctivitis, along with maculopapular rash which starts on** the face and migrates down to the trunk, **Koplick's spots are red macules with a white center found on the buccal mucosa,** but while these are pathognomonic they occur prior to the onset of the rash and typically resolve prior to the onset of the rash, so they **are often not present when the child presents,** note that measles can be life-threatening in immunocompromised children

vi) Treatment: supportive

vii) Resistance: not applicable

viii) Prophylaxis: a highly effective live-attenuated vaccine

b) Mumps Virus

i) Genome: single-stranded RNA

ii) Lab assays: serology

iii) Virulence factors: none significant

iv) Epidemiology: airborne transmission

v) Clinical Diseases: **flu-like prodrome leads in to acute onset of parotid swelling** (unilateral or bilateral), although typically self-limiting after a week or so, **some post-pubescent males can develop orchitis which can cause sterility if bilateral,** and rarely patients may develop aseptic meningitis

vi) Treatment: supportive

vii) Resistance: not applicable

viii) Prophylaxis: a highly effective live-attenuated vaccine

c) Parainfluenza Virus

i) Genome: single-stranded RNA

ii) Lab assays: none significant

iii) Virulence factors: none significant

iv) Epidemiology: airborne transmission

v) Clinical Diseases: presents in **children with Croup, a laryngotracheobronchitis typified by a dry, "barking cough"** and hoarse voice, can cause any URI in adults

      vi) Treatment: supportive, inhaled bronchodilators and inhaled, humidified air are helpful measures in patients with Croup

      vii) Resistance: not applicable

      viii) Prophylaxis: none

  d) Respiratory Syncytial Virus (RSV)

      i)   Genome: single-stranded RNA

      ii) Lab assays: Direct Fluorescent Antibody

      iii) Virulence factors: none significant

      iv) Epidemiology: airborne transmission

      v)   Clinical Diseases: mild URI in older children and adults, but can cause a **severe pneumonia in young children**, and is a common cause of Acute Respiratory Distress Syndrome in them

      vi) Treatment: ribavirin is used, but efficacy unclear

      vii) Resistance: not applicable

      viii) Prophylaxis: none

7) Rhabdovirus

  a) Rabies Virus

      i)   Genome: single-stranded RNA

      ii) Lab assays: **biopsy of infected neurons showing Negri bodies**

      iii) Virulence factors: binds to the acetylcholine receptor to mediate uptake into neurons

      iv) Epidemiology:

          a)) **Transmitted via saliva into bite by rabid animal**, cases are exceedingly rare in the US due to frequent vaccination of animals, but the **virus is common in bats and skunks** throughout the US and can occur in **canines near the US–Mexico border**

          b)) Following inoculation in the wound, the virus binds to peripheral neurons and is carried retrograde back to the CNS where it infects parts of the brain controlling aggression, making infected individuals prone to biting which can spread the virus to a new host

TABLE 28	**Summary of Encapsulated RNA Viruses**		
VIRUS	**TRANSMIS-SION**	**DISEASE**	**VACCINE?**
Coronavirus (positive polarity)			
Coronavirus	Airborne	Common cold	None
Flaviviruses (positive polarity)			
Dengue Virus	*Aedes* mosquito	Breakbone & hemorrhagic fever	None
Hepatitis C Virus	Blood	Hepatitis, cirrhosis, hepatocellular CA	None
Yellow Fever	*Aedes* mosquito	Hepatitis, hemorrhagic fever	Yes
Retroviruses (positive polarity)			
HIV	Body fluids, sex	Acute serovonversion syndrome, AIDS	No
HTLV	Body fluids, sex	T-cell leukemia/lymphoma and tropical spastic paraparesis, common in Japan and the Caribbean	No
Togaviruses (positive polarity)			
Encephaliti-des	Mosquito bite	Encephalitis	No
Rubella	Airborne, vertical	German measles, congenital defects	Yes
Arenaviruses (negative polarity)			
LCM Virus	Rodent exposure	Severe aseptic meningitis	No
Lassa Fever Virus	Rodent exposure	Hemorrhagic fever	No
Bunyaviruses (negative polarity)			
California Encephalitis Virus	Mosquitoes	Encephalitis	No
Hantavirus	Rodent droppings	ARDS	No

	TRANSMIS-		
VIRUS	**SION**	**DISEASE**	**VACCINE?**

TABLE 28 *Continued*

Deltavirus (negative polarity)

Hepatitis D Virus	Body fluids, sex	Hepatitis (in conjunction with HBV)	Yes*

Filoviruses (negative polarity)

Ebola- Marburg	Unknown	Hemorrhagic fever	No

Orthomyxoviruses (negative polarity)

Influenza	Airborne	The flu	Yes

Paramyxoviruses (negative polarity)

Measles	Airborne	Measles: cough, coryza, conjunctivitis	Yes
Mumps	Airborne	Mumps: parotid swelling, orchitis	Yes
Parainflu- enza Virus	Airborne	Croup: barking cough	No
Respiratory Syncytial Virus	Airborne	URI in older kids, pneumonia in younger	No

Rhabdovirus (negative polarity)

Rabies Virus	Animal bite	Confusion, hydrophobia, seizures, coma	Yes

*The HBV vaccine is effective against HDV because HBV is necessary for HDV to cause disease.

v) Clinical Diseases: within several weeks of bite (shorter time the closer the bite is to the head) the patient develops flu-like prodrome followed by acute onset of altered mental status, hypersalivation, and **painful spasms in the oropharynx on swallowing leading to the classic symptom of hydrophobia where a patient is afraid to swallow water due to the pain,** the disease inevitably progresses from seizures to coma, death is invariable

TABLE 29 Overall Summary of Viruses

	GENOME*	KEY WORD/PHRASES	VACCINE
Naked DNA Viruses			
Adenovirus	dsDNA	Pharyngoconjunctival fever, gastroenteritis	No
Human Papillomavirus	dsDNA	Warts, cervical cancer, fomite transmission	No
JC Polyomavirus	dsDNA	Encephalopathy (PML) in AIDS pts	No
BK Polyomavirus	dsDNA	Nephritis in kidney transplants	No
Parvovirus B19	ssDNA	Aplastic crisis in hemolysis pts, 5th dz in kids	No
Encapsulated DNA Viruses			
Hepatitis B Virus	dsDNA	10% of adults get chronic infection, 90% of vertically transmitted is chronic, tx with lamivudine or interferon-α	Yes
Cytomegalo-virus	dsDNA	HHV 5#, heterophile-negative mononucleosis in healthy people, severe hepatitis, pneumonia, retinitis in AIDS or organ transplant patients	No
Epstein-Barr Virus	dsDNA	HHV 4#, heterophile-positive mononucleosis	No
Herpes Simplex 1	dsDNA	HHV 1#, oral ulcers, conjunctivitis, meningitis	No
Herpes Simplex 2	dsDNA	HHV 2#, genital ulcers, meningitis	No
HHV 6 & 7#	dsDNA	Roseola infantum	No
HHV 8#	dsDNA	Kaposi' s sarcoma in AIDS pts	No
Varicella-Zoster Virus	dsDNA	HHV 3#, chicken pox and zoster (dermatomal pain and vesicular rash in elderly and sick)	Yes
Molluscum Poxvirus	dsDNA	Molluscum contagiosum in AIDS pts	No
Smallpox	dsDNA	Smallpox, eradicated from globe	Yes

TABLE 29 *Continued*

	GENOME*	KEY WORD/PHRASES	VACCINE
Naked RNA Viruses			
Hepatitis E	ss⊕ RNA	Hepatitis with high mortality in pregnancy	No
Norwalk	ss⊕ RNA	Gastroenteritis, often undercooked shellfish	No
Coxsackievirus	ss⊕ RNA	An enterovirus, causes multiple diseases including URI, serositis, myocarditis, Hand–Foot–Mouth dz, Herpangina, and meningitis	No
Echovirus	ss⊕ RNA	An enterovirus, causes URI and meningitis	No
Hepatitis A	ss⊕ RNA	Acute viral hepatitis	Yes
Polio	ss⊕ RNA	Rare pts get meningitis and full-blown polio	Yes
Rhinovirus	ss⊕ RNA	#1 cause of the common cold	No
Rotavirus	dsRNA	#1 cause diarrhea in the world, often age <2	No
Encapsulated RNA Viruses			
Coronavirus	ss⊕ RNA	#2 cause of the common cold	No
Dengue	ss⊕ RNA	Breakbone fever (myalgias and arthralgias so severe it feels like bones are breaking)	No
Hepatitis C	ss⊕ RNA	90% of infected have chronic dz, treat with combination ribavirin and interferon-α	No
Yellow Fever	ss⊕ RNA	Severe hepatitis and hemorrhagic fever	Yes
Human Immunodeficiency	ss⊕ RNA	p24 antigen present during seroconversion when ELISA is negative, kills CD4 T-cells, death from infection or malignancy	No
Human T-cell Leukemia	ss⊕ RNA	Causes T-cell leukemia and lymphoma, and tropical spastic paraparesis, highest prevalence in Japan and the Caribbean	No

TABLE 29	*Continued*		
	GENOME*	**KEY WORD/PHRASES**	**VACCINE**
Encephalitis	ss⊕ RNA	Transmitted by mosquitoes, often fatal	No
Rubella	ss⊕ RNA	German measles = fever and rash, self-lmtd	Yes
Lymphocytic Choriomeningitis	ss-RNA	Severe aseptic meningitis, may be fatal	No
Lassa Fever	ss-RNA	Hemorrhagic fever	No
California Encephalitis	ss-RNA	Transmitted by mosquito	No
Hantavirus	ss-RNA	Exposure to rodents in rural desert areas, causes rapidly progressive ARDS	No
Hepatitis D	ss-RNA	Only infective in the presence of HBV	Yes^ψ
Ebola-Marburg	ss-RNA	Hemorrhagic fever, up to 90% mortality	No
Influenza	ss-RNA	Striking myalgias and fever, no GI symptoms	Yes
Measles	ss-RNA	Cough, coryza, conjunctivitis, maculopapular rash, Koplick's spots	Yes
Mumps	ss-RNA	Rash, parotid swelling, orchitis	Yes
Parainfluenza	ss-RNA	Croup, hoarse voice and "barking cough"	No
Respiratory Syncytial	ss-RNA	URI in older kids, pneumonia in younger kids	No
Rabies	ss-RNA	Binds to acetylcholine receptor, migrates to CNS so bites closer to head cause disease more rapidly, classic symptom is hydrophobia where pt fears drinking water due to painful spasms in oropharynx when swallowing	Yes

*ds = double stranded, ss = single stranded, ⊕ = positive polarity, − = negative polarity; #HHV = Human Herpes Virus; ψHBV vaccine is effective as HDV only causes dz in the presence of HBV.

vi) Treatment: supportive once disease onsets

vii) Resistance: not applicable

viii) Prophylaxis:

   a)) Pre-exposure prophylaxis is via rabies vaccine, which should be given to anyone in contact with wild animals

   b)) **Post-exposure prophylaxis is via both administration of rabies vaccine and rabies immune globulin given concurrently but at different sites to prevent neutralization of the vaccine by the antibody**

VI. ANTIBIOTICS

A. Bacterial Agents

1. Penicillins

   a. Mechanism: **inhibits bacterial cell wall synthesis** by blocking the **transpeptidase**-dependent cross-linkage of peptidoglycan

   b. Resistance: several mechanisms described

      1) **β-lactamase production**: many bacteria express β-lactamase, an enzyme that cleaves open the 5-membered β-lactam ring in penicillins, inactivating them—this can be overcome by adding a β-lactamase inhibitor to the penicillin, which protects the penicillin from the bacterial β-lactamase

      2) Altered penicillin binding proteins (PBPs): some bacteria have mutated penicillin binding targets (the transpeptidases), this is the mechanism for Methicillin-Resistant *Staphylococcus aureus* (MRSA)

   c. Toxicities: hypersensitivity reactions (including anaphylaxis) common, can also see leukopenia and can induce autoimmune hemolytic anemia

   d. Cidal/Static: cidal for actively dividing bacteria

   e. Coverage:

      1) Penicillin: good *Strep* coverage and **good for oral anaerobes**, good for strep throat, oral/dental infections, syphilis, bad for gram negatives

2) Aminopenicillins (e.g., ampicillin): addition of amino group **adds coverage for Enterococcus and Listeria,** and some gram negatives

3) Addition of β-lactamase inhibitor (e.g., ampicillin + sulbactam): **markedly expands coverage,** including most *Enterococcus,* most *Staphylococcus,* most *Streptococcus,* most community acquired gram negative rods (but not nosocomials like *Pseudomonas*), most anaerobes (including abdominal anaerobes)

4) Penicillinase-resistant penicillins (e.g., oxacillin): **specifically designed to hit Staphylococcus,** covers all *Staphylococcus* except those with altered penicillin binding proteins (so-called Methicillin Resistant Staphylococci or MRSA) at the expense of losing some coverage on *Streptococcus* and losing all coverage on *Enterococcus* and gram negatives

5) Ureidopenicillins (e.g., piperacillin): **designed for expanded gram negative coverage,** covers gram positives per aminopenicillins, but **also covers nosocomial gram negatives** like many strains of *Pseudomonas*—note that **addition of β-lactamase inhibitor (e.g., piperacillin-tazobactam) creates an incredibly powerful drug which covers virtually all gram positives (except MRSA and some Enterococcus), virtually all gram negatives including most Pseudomonas, and virtually all anaerobes**

2. Cephalosporins

a. Mechanism: like penicillins, **inhibits bacterial cell wall synthesis** by blocking the transpeptidase-dependent cross-linkage of peptidoglycan

b. Resistance: two major mechanisms

1) β-lactamase production: although cephalosporins have a 6-membered ring instead of the 5-membered β-lactam ring, β-lactamase enzymes still destroy cephalosporins

2) Altered penicillin binding proteins

c. Toxicities: hypersensitivity reactions less common than penicillins and **only 15% cross-reactivity between penicillin allergy and cephalosporin allergy,** cephalosporins also can cause biliary sludging. Can inhibit risk uptake in GI and cause coagulation abnormalities

d. Cidal/Static: cidal for actively dividing bacteria

e. Coverage:

1) 1st generation (e.g., cefazolin): very good *Staphylococcus* and *Streptococcus* coverage, makes them **good for skin infections**, and hits community acquired gram negatives (e.g., *E. coli*) so good for UTIs

2) 2nd generation (e.g., cefuroxime): better *Streptococcus* coverage but worse *Staphylococcus* coverage, better community acquired gram negative coverage, **good for outpatient community acquired pneumonia**, some have very good anaerobic coverage (e.g., cefotetan)

3) 3rd generation: difficult to assess by class, two specifics to know

   a) Ceftriaxone: **best *Streptococcus* coverage of all, loses most *Staphylococcus* coverage, good community acquired gram negatives but does not hit nosocomial gram negatives,** 1st line for meningitis and in-patient community acquired pneumonia

   b) Ceftazidime: **loses all gram positive coverage but excellent gram negative coverage including most nosocomials including *Pseudomonas*, used for nosocomial infections**

3. Carbapenems

   a. Mechanism: like penicillins, inhibits bacterial cell wall synthesis by blocking the transpeptidase-dependent cross-linkage of peptidoglycan

   b. Resistance: β-lactamases don't work well against carbapenems so this is not a mechanism of resistance, however altered penicillin binding proteins still a problem

   c. Toxicities: seizures

   d. Cidal/Static: cidal for actively dividing bacteria

   e. Coverage: imipenem and meropenum are very similar except meropenum doesn't cause seizures, both probably the broadest spectrum coverage available in any one drug, cover most gram positives, most gram negatives including *Pseudomonas*, and most anaerobes

4. Monobactams

   a. Mechanism: like penicillins, inhibits bacterial cell wall synthesis by blocking the transpeptidase-dependent cross-linkage of peptidoglycan

   b. Resistance: β-lactamases don't work well against monobactams so this is not a mechanism of resistance, however altered penicillin binding proteins still a problem

   c. Toxicities: minimal, no cross-reactivity to penicillins

   d. Cidal/Static: cidal for actively dividing bacteria

   e. Coverage: one drug, aztreonam, **covers most gram negatives including nosocomials like *Pseudomonas*, but loses all anaerobic and gram positive coverage**

5. Glycopeptide

   a. Mechanism: like penicillins, **inhibits bacterial cell wall synthesis**, but unlike penicillins they **act by binding to D-alanine-D-alanine subunits of the cell wall** and preventing their insertion into the cell wall

   b. Resistance: all gram negatives are intrinsically resistant, gram positive resistance is unusual but can occur via a variety of mechanisms

   c. Toxicities: azotemia, "Red Man syndrome" (skin flushing)

   d. Cidal/Static: static

   e. Coverage: vancomycin is the major parenteral version (teicoplanin is not yet approved in the US), bacitracin is a topical version, vancomycin **covers all gram positive organisms** except Vancomycin Resistant *Enterococcus* (VRE) and very rarely reported isolates of Vancomycin Resistant *Staphylococcus aureus* (VRSA)

6. Aminoglycosides

   a. Mechanism: **binds to 30S subunit of bacterial ribosome, blocking protein synthesis initiation and causing misreading of the mRNA code**

   b. Resistance: several major mechanisms described

     1) Altered uptake of the drug

     2) Bacterial enzymes stick acetyl groups on aminoglycosides, modifying the drugs' structures, thereby inactivating them

     3) Mutations in bacterial ribosomes, blocking the drugs' ability to bind to their targets

     4) Anaerobes are intrinsically resistant, as aminoglycosides require an oxidative environment to be transported into the cell

   c. Toxicities: **renal tubular damage** and **ototoxicity** are the most prominent toxicities

    d. Cidal/Static: cidal

    e. Coverage: streptomycin is rarely used, gentamicin is most commonly used, **covers virtually all gram negatives, including nosocomials** like *Pseudomonas*, also **acts synergistically with cell-wall inhibitors** (e.g., penicillins) against gram positives (the cell-wall inhibitors open pores in the cell wall, allowing the bulky aminoglycoside to pass into the cell)

7. Tetracyclines

    a. Mechanism: **binds to 30S subunit of bacterial ribosome, blocking the acceptor site for the incoming aminoacyl-tRNA**, thereby inhibiting protein synthesis

    b. Resistance: due to decreased uptake or actual efflux of the drug from the bacteria mediated by a pump protein

    c. Toxicities: discoloration of teeth in children

    d. Cidal/Static: static

    e. Coverage: doxycycline is by far the most commonly used, **excellent coverage for atypical, intracellular organisms**

8. Chloramphenicol

    a. Mechanism: **binds to the 50S subunit of bacterial ribosome, blocking the action of peptidyltransferase** which inhibits formation of the peptide bond

    b. Resistance: most common mechanism is acetylation of the drug, thereby inactivating it, can also be due to decreased drug uptake

    c. Toxicities:

        1) Dose-dependent aplastic anemia, reversible with cessation of the drug

        2) **Idiosyncratic aplastic anemia, not reversible after drug cessation** and not related to total dose of drug given, **interestingly it has only been reported after oral administration of the drug**, never after intravenous administration

        3) **Gray-baby syndrome is due to uncoupling of oxidative phosphorylation** in the myocardium in infants, causing cyanosis and shock

    d. Cidal/Static: static

    e. Coverage: only one drug in the class, very broad spectrum activity, including gram positives, many

community-acquired gram negative rods, atypical/intracel-
lular organisms, and many anaerobes, but not considered
1st line for any infections in the developed world

9. Macrolides

   a. Mechanism: **binds to 50S subunit of bacterial ribosome
   and blocks translocation of amino acids,** interfering with
   protein synthesis

   b. Resistance: due to decreased cell uptake, enzymatic inacti-
   vation of the drugs, or mutations affecting the drugs'
   binding site on the ribosome

   c. Toxicities: **GI upset with nausea and vomiting is very
   common with erythromycin,** drug interactions with
   agents metabolized by cytochrome P450 (such as antihistamines) **causes QT prolongation which can lead to
   Torsades de Pointes**

   d. Cidal/Static: static

   e. Coverage:

      1) 1st generation: erythromycin is the old stand-by, covers
      Streptococcus spp. and atypicals but has no gram nega-
      tive coverage, and is still used by some for community
      acquired pneumonia because it covers many
      Streptococcus pneumonia strains as well as atypicals such
      as *Mycoplasma* and *Legionella*, **erythromycin is also typi-
      cally the drug of choice to treat penicillin-sensitive
      infections in penicillin-allergic patients**

      2) 2nd generation: clarithromycin and azithromycin are
      much better tolerated (less GI adverse effects), have
      excellent *Streptococcus* and atypical coverage, but still
      minimal gram negative coverage, and are considered
      first line for outpatient community acquired pneumo-
      nia (superior *Streptococcus pneumonia* and atypical cov-
      erage, including for *Legionella*), *H. pylori* infection, and
      Mycobacterium avium intracellulare

10. Lincosamide

    a. Mechanism: **binds to 50S subunit of bacterial ribosome
    and blocks formation of peptide bond**

    b. Resistance: due to mutations altering the drug's binding
    site on the bacterial ribosomes

    c. Toxicities: **major risk is the triggering of *Clostridium diffi-
    cile*** infection by wiping out the enteric flora, occurring in
    up to 10% of patients

    d. Cidal/Static: cidal for gram positive cocci, static for anaerobes

    e. Coverage: clindamycin is the major drug in the class, **first line for anaerobic infections in the lung or oropharynx,** good 2nd line agent for bowel anaerobes (behind metronidazole), also quite good activity against both *Streptococcus* and *Staphylococcus spp.*, making it useful for cellulitis (2nd line behind cephalosporins)

11. Streptogramins

    a. Mechanism: **bind to the 50S subunit of bacterial ribosomes,** inhibiting protein synthesis

    b. Resistance: gram negatives and *Enterococcus faecalis* intrinsically resistant

    c. Toxicities: severe thrombophlebitis, requires central venous access

    d. Cidal/Static: static

    e. Coverage: quinupristin/dalfopristin (Synercid®) is the only drug used in this class, **covers most gram positives, including VRE** (but not *E. faecalis*, fortunately most VRE is *E. faecium*), **and MRSA**

12. Oxazolidinone

    a. Mechanism: **binds to the 50S subunit of bacterial ribosomes,** inhibiting protein synthesis by a unique mechanism, that is it **prevents union of the 50S and 30S subunits into the 70S pre-initiation complex,** thereby stopping protein synthesis before it ever begins

    b. Resistance: thus far none described

    c. Toxicities: anemia and thrombocytopenia

    d. Cidal/Static: static

    e. Coverage: linezolid is the only drug in this class, newly approved by the FDA in 2000, **covers essentially all gram positive organisms, including VRE and MRSA**

13. Fluoroquinolones

    a. Mechanism: **blocks activity of DNA gyrase,** which unwinds bacterial DNA during genomic replication

    b. Resistance: due to mutations in DNA gyrase, making it resistant to the drugs' activity

c. Toxicities: may cause bone or joint disease in children (only convincingly demonstrated in experimental animals), including tendon rupture

d. Cidal/Static: cidal

e. Coverage:

1) **Ciprofloxacin has the best gram negative activity in the class,** best *Pseudomonas* coverage at expense of minimal gram positive coverage, has excellent atypical coverage—excellent drug for kidney (e.g., pyelonephritis), GU (e.g., prostatitis), bowel (e.g., gastroenteritis), & bone (e.g., osteomyelitis)

2) **Levofloxacin/ofloxacin cover *Streptococcus* well but not *Staphylococcus*,** cover gram negatives but not as well as cipro, and have **excellent atypical coverage,** useful for same infxns as cipro, but also pneumonia

3) Moxifloxacin/gatifloxacin have extended *Strep* and *Staph* coverage

14. Bactrim (trimethoprim/sulfamethoxazole)

a. Mechanism: the **trimethoprim blocks dihydrofolate reductase,** inhibiting generation of folate, while **sulfamethoxazole** acts earlier in the folate pathway by acting as a **structural analogue for para-aminobenzoic acid** (PABA), a folate precursor

b. Resistance: mutations in the folate synthetic pathway and in the enzyme targets

c. Toxicities: allergic reactions common, ranging from rash to anaphylaxis, rarely folate deficiency may result after prolonged drug intake causing megaloblastic bone marrow suppression

d. Cidal/Static: cidal

e. Coverage: Bactrim is a synergistic combination of its two components, good coverage for *Streptococcus*, covers some *Staphylococcus*, good coverage for community acquired gram negative rods (but not nosocomial), **its concentration in the kidney, urine, and prostate make it ideal for uncomplicated UTIs, kidney infections, and GU infections,** and it can be used for community acquired pneumonia, it is also highly active against *Pneumocystic carinii* and *Toxoplasma*, and is used both therapeutically and prophylactically against these organisms

TABLE 30	Summary of Antibacterial Antibiotics			
CLASS (EXAMPLE)	**TARGET**	**PROCESS INHIBITED**	**TOXICITY**	**KEY COVERAGE**
Penicillin (PCN)	Transpeptidase	Cell wall synthesis	Allergic	*Strep*, oral anaerobes
Aminopenicillin (ampicillin)	Transpeptidase	Cell wall synthesis	Allergic	*Enterococcus, Listeria*
β-lactamase inhibitor + amp (amp/sulbactam)	Transpeptidase	Cell wall synthesis	Allergic	GPC, GNR, anaerobes but not nosocomials
Penicillinase-resistant PCN (oxacillin)	Transpeptidase	Cell wall synthesis	Allergic	*Staphylococcus* only
Ureidopenicillin (piperacillin)	Transpeptidase	Cell wall synthesis	Allergic	GPC, GNR, anaerobes, & nosocomials
1° Cephalosporin (cefazolin)	Transpeptidase	Cell wall synthesis	Allergic	*Staph/Strep*, some GNR
2° Cephalosporin (cefuroxime)	Transpeptidase	Cell wall synthesis	Allergic	Better *Strep*, better GNR, worse *Staph*
3° Cephalosporin (ceftriaxone/ ceftazidime)	Transpeptidase	Cell wall synthesis	Allergic	*Strep* & GNR, nosocomial (ceftazidime)
Carbapenum (imipenem)	Transpeptidase	Cell wall synthesis	Seizure	Broad coverage including nosocomials
Monobactam (aztreonam)	Transpeptidase	Cell wall synthesis	Minimal	GNR including nosocomials
Glycopeptides (vancomycin)	D-alanine-D-alanine	Cell wall synthesis	Allergic	All GPC
Aminoglycoside (gentamicin)	30S ribosome	Protein synthesis	Renal and ototoxic	GNR including nosocomials
Tetracyclines (doxycycline)	50S ribosome	Protein synthesis	Bone/teeth coloration	Atypicals

TABLE 30	*Continued*			
CLASS (EXAMPLE)	**TARGET**	**PROCESS INHIBITED**	**TOXICITY**	**KEY COVERAGE**
Chloramphenicol	50S ribosome	Protein synthesis	Bone marrow	Broad but not nosocomials
Macrolide (erythromycin)	50S ribosome	Protein synthesis	GI upset	*Strep* and atypicals
lincosamide (clindamycin)	50S ribosome	Protein synthesis	*C. difficile*	GPC, excellent for anaerobes
Streptogramin (Synercid®)	50S ribosome	Protein synthesis	Thrombophlebitis	VRE and MRSA
Oxazolidinone (linezolid)	50S ribosome	Protein synthesis	Anemia	All GPC
Fluoroquinolones (ciprofloxacin)	DNA gyrase	DNA replication	Bone/joint damage	*Strep*, GNR, nosocomials, atypicals
Bactrim	PABA/ dihydrofolate reductase	Folate synthesis	Allergic	GPC, GNR, protozoa
Metronidazole	Unclear	Anaerobic metabolism	Minimal	1st line anaerobes
Rifamycins (rifampin)	RNA polymerase	RNA transcription	Red urine & tears	GPC, GNR, atypicals
Isoniazid	Unclear	Mycolic acid synthesis	Hepatic, deplete B6	*Mycobacteria*

15. Metronidazole

    a. Mechanism: exact target unclear, but it **poisons anaerobic metabolism**

    b. Resistance: unusual, may be due to slow drug uptake

    c. Toxicities: minimal

    d. Cidal/Static: cidal

    e. Coverage: only the one drug in the class, **by far the most effective agent for all bowel anaerobes**, should be used for all biliary, hepatic, and bowel infections and all abscesses in the body, **first line for amebic abscesses**

16. Rifamycins

    a. Mechanism: **inhibit RNA polymerase**

    b. Resistance: **resistance very commonly develops during monotherapy**, requiring that rifamycins always be given in combination with a 2nd agent, mechanism is mutation of bacterial RNA polymerase

    c. Toxicities: turns body secretions red

    d. Cidal/Static: cidal

    e. Coverage: broad spectrum activity when combined with a second agent, 1st line as part of combination chemotherapy for TB, useful as combination therapy for endocarditis or osteomyelitis due to **excellent tissue penetration**, used for close-contact prophylaxis in meninigitis due to good salivary penetration, rifampin and rifabutin have similar activities

17. Isoniazid

    a. Mechanism: somehow **inhibits mycolic acid synthesis**

    b. Resistance: develops spontaneously in bacterial chromosomes at a certain set rate, so resistance develops during monotherapy if the organism burden in the patient is high enough to make it statistically possible

    c. Toxicities: **risk of fulminant hepatic toxicity, also commonly depletes vitamin B6**

    d. Cidal/Static: cidal

    e. Coverage: the only drug in the class, extremely effective for TB, also effective against other mycobacteria

B. Fungal Agents

1. Polyenes

    a. Mechanism: **binds to ergosterol in the fungal cell membrane**, punching holes in the membrane

    b. Resistance: not seen clinically

    c. Toxicities: extremely toxic agents, very poorly tolerated by patients due to **severe rigors and malaise, invariably causes dose-dependent renal insufficiency, renal tubular acidosis with potassium and magnesium wasting, and bone marrow suppression**

    d. Cidal/Static: cidal

e. Coverage: nystatin is only used orally and is not absorbed, so it is useful for oropharyngeal or esophageal thrush, while **amphotericin is the mainstay of severe, invasive fungal infections, and should be used for all fungal infections in unstable or neutropenic patients,** liposomal formulations are now available which are less toxic, allowing increasing doses to be administered

2. Azoles

   a. Mechanism: **inhibits ergosterol synthesis by disrupting the cytochrome P450 pathway**

   b. Resistance: some species are intrinsically resistant due to altered P450 enzymes (e.g., *Candida krusei*), resistance is an as-of-yet uncommon but definitely increasing problem

   c. Toxicities: GI intolerance, cholestasis, hepatitis are the most common

   d. Cidal/Static: static

   e. Coverage: although miconazole and clotrimazole are used topically, fluconazole and itraconazole are really the only two azoles still used for invasive disease, **fluconazole has excellent *Candida*, *Cryptococcus*, and *Coccidioides* coverage (that is, it hits yeast very well), but it doesn't cover molds at all,** whereas itraconazole has reasonable *Aspergillus* **coverage but is less well tolerated than fluconazole,** so use fluconazole for all yeast infections and itraconazole for *Aspergillus*

REVIEW QUESTIONS

1. A fifty-year-old man complains for several days of a cough productive of greenish sputum. He has a fever of 101°F, an infiltrate on CXR, and a positive sputum culture. What laboratory test pattern is the most likely for the organism growing from his sputum?

   a) GPC in clusters, coagulase positive

   b) GPC in chains, β-hemolytic

   c) GPC in pairs, quellung positive

   d) GPC in chains, CAMP factor positive

   e) GPC in pairs, resistant to hypertonic saline

2. Gram stain of a clinical specimen reveals gram positive cocci in pairs and chains. Laboratory testing reveals resistance to bile, hydrolysis of esculin, and resistance to hypertonic saline. Susceptibility testing reveals resistance to penicillin and vancomycin. What antibiotic would you recommend for coverage?

   a) Ampicillin

   b) Ampicillin + sulbactam

   c) Gentamicin

   d) Imepenum

   e) Linezolid

3. Match the following gastrointestinal toxidromes with their causative organism:

   1) *E. coli* O157:H7   a) Reheated fried rice

   2) *Staph. aureus*   b) Onset of sx at 6 hr after consumption

   3) *Bacillus cereus*   c) Onset 16 hr after eating reheated food

   4) *Vibrio cholera*   d) ADP-ribosylation of G-protein in intesintal cells

   5) *C. perfringens*   e) Hemolytic-uremic syndrome

4. A sixty-year-old alcoholic male is brought into the emergency room after being found down on the street. The patient is confused but not tremulous. His alcohol level is zero. He is febrile and tachycardic, and has meningismus on exam. His lumbar puncture shows a thousand white cells, consistent with meningitis. What antibiotics should be started for this patient and why?

   a) Ceftriaxone to cover for *Streptococcus pneumonia*, *Hemophilus*, and *Neisseria meningitidis*

   b) Ceftazadime to cover for *Pseudomonas*

   c) Ceftriaxone and gentamicin to cover for *S. pneumonia*, *Hemophilus*, *Neisseria*, and *Listeria*

   d) Ampicillin and ceftriaxone to cover for *S. pneumonia*, *Hemophilus*, *Neisseria*, and *Listeria*

   e) Ceftriaxone to cover *S. pneumonia*, *Hemophilus*, and *Neisseria*, and gentamicin for synergistic coverage for *Streptococcus agalactiae*

5. Match the following immunodeficiencies with the organisms to which they impart susceptibility (each immunodeficiency can only be used once!):

   1) Splenectomy
   2) CD4 count <200
   3) Neutropenia
   4) C6 deficiency
   5) Renal transplant

   a) BK Polyomavirus
   b) *Aspergillus* dissemination
   c) *Neisseria meningitidis*
   d) *Streptococcus pneumonia*
   e) *Pneumocystic carinii*

6. The following are defining characteristics of Enterobacteriaceae **except**:

   a) Facultative anaerobes

   b) Ferment lactose

   c) Oxidase negative

   d) Ferment glucose

   e) Reduce nitrates to nitrites

7. Match the following diseases to their most common etiological agent (each bacteria can be used once, more than once or not at all):

   1) Meningitis in adults
   2) Community acquired pneumonia
   3) Urinary tract infection
   4) Gastroenteritis in the US
   5) Meningitis in neonates

   a) *E. coli*
   b) *Campylobacter*
   c) *Streptococcus pneumonia*
   d) *Streptococcus agalactiae*
   e) *Staphylococcus aureus*

8. Match the following organisms with special requirements for culture:

   1) *Hemophilus influenza*
   2) *Corynebacterium*
   3) *Neisseria gonorrhoeae*
   4) *Legionella*
   5) TB

   a) Iron and cysteine supplements
   b) Lowenstein–Jensen medium
   c) Tellurite agar
   d) Thayer–Martin agar
   e) Factor V & Factor X

9. Match the following causes of community acquired

pneumonia with its special characteristics:

1) *Staph. aureus* a) Diarrhea, hyponatremia, very high LDH

2) *Acinetobacter* b) Lung abscesses following aspiration pneumonia

3) *Klebsiella* c) Follows antecendent influenza

4) *Legionella* d) Nosocomial pneumonia in ICU patients on ventilators

5) *Bacteroides* e) "currant-jelly" hemoptysis, often in diabetics or alcoholics

10. Match the following zoonotic organisms with their risks for transmission?

1) *Brucella* a) Dog bite

2) *Francisella* b) Milk and farm animals

3) *Pasteurella* c) Flea

4) *Yersinia pestis* d) Tick

11. Match the following patients with the appropriate PPD diameter for treating with isoniazid (letters can be used more than once):

1) A thirty-year-old homeless man a) 5 mm

2) A twenty-five-year-old healthy male b) 10 mm

3) A forty-year-old healthy male with no risks c) 15 mm

4) A sixty-year-old pt with old dz on CXR d) No tx

5) A forty-five-year-old male with AIDS

12. Which of the following spirochetes does **not** cause significant CNS disease?

a) *Treponema pallidum*

b) *Borrelia burgdorferi*

c) *Borrelia recurrentis*

d) *Leptospira*

13. Which of the following is not a risk factor for invasive candidiasis?

    a) AIDS

    b) Neutropenia

    c) Central venous catheters

    d) Parenteral nutrition

    e) Laparotomy

14. Match the following risk factors with the appropriate fungus:

1) Pigeon droppings	a) *Histoplasma*
2) Spelunking	b) *Sporothrix*
3) Antibiotics	c) *Rhizopus*
4) Serum pH 7.20	d) *Candida*
5) Rose bushes	e) *Cryptococcus*

15. Which of the following protozoa commonly causes abscesses?

    a) *Cryptosporidium*

    b) *Entamoeba*

    c) *Giardia*

    d) *Trichomonas*

16. Match the following invasive protozoa with their appropriate vectors:

1) *Leishmania*	a) Reduviid bug
2) *Plasmodium*	b) Sandfly
3) *Trypanosoma cruzi*	c) Tsetse fly
4) *Trypanosoma gambiense*	d) *Anopholes* mosquito

17. Which of the following statements regarding *Plasmodium* infections is **not** true?

    a) *P. falciparum* malaria is phenotypically the most severe

    b) Tertian fevers occur every 48 hr

    c) Quartan fever can be treated with chloroquine alone

    d) Tertian fever can be treated with primaquine alone

    e) Resistance to quinines is becoming a worldwide problem

18. Match the following helminths to the exposures most likely to result in their infection (exposures may be used more than once):

    1) *Diphyllobothrium*   a) Raw crab meat

    2) *Echinococcus*   b) Raw pork

    3) *Taenia saginata*   c) Raw fish

    4) *Taenia solium*   d) Dogs and sheep

    5) *Clonorchis sinensis*   e) Raw beef

    6) *Paragonimus westermani*

    7) *Trichinella spiralis*

19. Which of the following statements is **false**?

    a) Hookworms are the leading cause of iron deficiency anemia worldwide

    b) *Ascaris* is the most common helminthic infection worldwide

    c) *Enterobius* is the most common helminthic infection in the United States of America

    d) *Trichiuris* causes rectal prolapse

    e) Prominent eosinophilia occurs in all parasitic infections

20. Match the following viruses to the diseases they cause:

    1) Adenovirus   a) Roseola infantum

    2) JC polyomavirus   b) Heterophile negative mononucleosis

    3) Parvovirus B19   c) Breakbone fever

    4) Cytomegalovirus   d) Kaposi's sarcoma

    5) HHV 6   e) Herpangina

    6) HHV 8   f) Progressive multifocal leukoencephalopathy

    7) Coxsackievirus   g) Tropical spastic paraparesis

    8) Dengue Virus   h) 5th disease, erythema infectiosum

    9) HTLV   i) Pharyngoconjunctival fever

21. Which of the following statements regarding Hepatitis B Virus is **false**?

a) Hepatitis B Virus e antigen titers correlate with infectivity of the patient

b) The most common mode of transmission worldwide is vertical

c) The "window period" is when the Hepatitis B Virus surface antigen is negative but the surface antibody test is positive

d) Hepatitis B Virus has a reverse transcriptase

e) Whereas Hepatitis B Surface Antibody correlates with immunity to infection the Hepatitis B Core Antibody is not protective

22. Match the following antibiotics with the biochemical step they inhibit:

1) Penicillin	a) Amino acid translocation
2) Gentamicin	b) Dihydrofolate reductase
3) Doxycycline	c) Mycolic acid synthesis
4) Chloramphenicol	d) Peptidyltransferase
5) Erythromycin	e) Formation of 70S
6) Clindamycin	f) RNA polymerase
7) Linezolid	g) Proper reading of mRNA codons
8) Ciprofloxacin	h) Transpeptidase
9) Bactrim®	i) Aminoacyl-tRNA binding
10) Rifampin	j) Peptide bond formation
11) Isoniazid	k) DNA gyrase

ANSWERS

1. **c)** *Streptococcus pneumonia* is the most common cause of community acquired pneumonia. *S. pneumonia* is gram positive and often described as *"diplococcus,"* meaning pairs of cocci, although it can also grow in chains (so "pairs and chains" is often seen). *S. pneumonia* is α-hemolytic, not β-hemolytic, and it has a prominent polysaccharide capsule which causes the quellung test to be positive. GPC in clusters refers to *Staphylococcus*, and the positive coagulase test would identify

S. aureus. β-hemolytic GPC in chains could be any of the "grouped" *Streptococci* (e.g., Group A, Group B, etc.). CAMP factor identifies Group B Strep, and GPC resistant to hypertonic saline identifies *Enterococcus.*

2. **e)** Gram positive cocci in pairs and chains resistant to bile that hydrolyzes esculin could be either *Streptococcus bovis* or *Enterococcus.* The resistance to hypertonic saline identifies the organism as *Enterococcus,* and the resistance to vancomycin identifies Vancomycin Resitant *Enterococcus* (VRE). As the VRE is also resistant to penicillin (which is often the case), linezolid (or quinupristin/dalfopristin, which wasn't one of the choices) must be used.

3. **1-e, 2-b, 3-a, 4-d, 5-c.** *S. aureus* exotoxin causes nausea, vomiting, and diarrhea within 8 hr of consumption of contaminated food. *Bacillus cereus* also causes rapid onset of symptoms, typically within 4 hr of consumption, although a longer incubation can also be seen. The classic buzz words for *B. cereus* gastroenteritis is the reheating of fried rice, which causes bacterial endospores to activate. In contrast *Clostridium perfringens* gastroenteritis typically occurs 8–16 hr after food consumption. *E. coli* O157:H7 secretes a Shiga-like toxin which can cause a severe inflammatory gastroenteritis, and in children can cause the hemolytic-uremic syndrome. *Vibrio cholera* toxin ADP-ribosylates a G-protein linked to an ion channel, allowing constant secretion of fluid and salt into the gut. This results in a secretory diarrhea.

4. **d)** The key to this question is the presence of meningitis in a compromised host. Specifically, alcoholism is associated with an increased susceptibility to *Listeria* meningitis (as is, for example, diabetes or any other chronic, debilitating illness). Ceftriaxone is empiric therapy of choice for all community acquired meningitis, but it does not cover *Listeria.* In general aminopenicillins, such as ampicillin, are the best coverage for *Listeria,* and must be added in this case.

5. **1-d, 2-e, 3-b, 4-c, 5-a.** Splenectomy results in relative suppression of antibody responses to blood-born infections. For microbes with anti-phagocytic polysaccharide capsules antibody production is key to host protection, as the antibody opsonizes the otherwise non-phagocytosable organism. Thus, splenectomy makes hosts susceptible to bacteremia caused by microbes with polysaccharide capsules, of which *S. pneumonia* is the most common example. AIDS patients with CD4 counts less than 200 are at markedly increased risk for developing *Pneumocystis* pneumonia. Neutropenia is the major risk factor for developing disseminated fungal

infections, particularly for *Aspergillus* and *Candida*, but also for *Mucor* and others. Deficiencies in the late components of the complement cascade (C5–C9), impart susceptibility to *Neisseria* infections. Renal transplant patients can develop nephritis from the BK Polyomavirus.

6. **b)** Enterobacteriaceae are all facultative anaerobes that ferment glucose, reduce nitrates to nitrites, and are oxidase negative. Only some (e.g., *E. coli, Enterobacter,* and *Klebsiella*) ferment lactose.

7. **1-c, 2-c, 3-a, 4-b, 5-d.** *Streptococcus pneumonia* is the most common cause of community acquired pneumonia and meningitis in adults in the United States. *Campylobacter* is the most common cause of invasive gastroenteritis in the United States, while *E. coli* is the most common cause of urinary tract infections. Group B strep is the number one cause of meningitis in neonates.

8. **1-e, 2-c, 3-d, 4-a, 5-b.**

9. **1-c, 2-d, 3-e, 4-a, 5-b.** *S. aureus* is a very uncommon cause of community acquired pneumonia. It occurs in two major settings: as a post-viral bacterial process or due to seeding of the lungs caused by *Staphylococcal* bacteremia. *Acinetobacter* is only seen in the nosocomial setting, typically in patients on ventilators. *Klebsiella* causes a necrotic lung process leading to prominent hemoptysis with thick, bloody mucous, described as "currant jelly." *Legionella* causes severe pneumonia associated with diarrhea, hyponatremia, and very high LDH. *Bacteroides* is an obligate anaerobe. The only time it can exist in the lung is in a polymicrobial abscess where the oxygen is utilized by facultative anaerobes.

10. **1-b, 2-d, 3-a, 4-c.** *Pasteurella* is typically transmitted from an animal bite, usually dog or cat. *Yersinia* is transmitted by fleas which have fed on rodents, while *Francisella* is spread by ticks having fed on rabbits or other mammals. *Brucella* is transmitted during contact with farm animals.

11. **1-b, 2-c, 3-c, 4-a, 5-a.** Patients with "high risk" for TB, including those with HIV, those in contact with people who have active disease, those with debilitating illnesses (such as renal failure or cancer), and those with evidence of old TB on CXR, should receive INH therapy if their PPDs are ≥5 mm. People with risk factors such as homelessness, imprisonment, immigration from high-risk areas (such as Latin America and Asia), and employment in health care should be treated if their PPDs are ≥10 mm. Healthy adults with no risk factors should be treated if they have PPDs ≥15 mm. In the past, these latter

patients would not have received INH if they were over 35 yr old. However, the updated guidelines from 2000 no longer take age into account for the decision to give INH. If you place a PPD and it is positive, the patient should be treated. On the other hand, the guidelines recommend not placing PPDs on elderly people without TB risks.

12. **c)** Syphilis (*T. pallidum*), Lyme disease (*B. burgdoreferi*), and Weil's disease (*Leptospira*) all cause prominent aseptic meningitis. *B. recurrentis* causes undulating fevers with lymphadenopathy.

13. **a)** For unclear reasons, AIDS patients get oral-mucosal candidiasis, but not invasive disease. Each of the other factors, along with broad spectrum antibiotics, are risks for invasive candidiasis. Any GI surgery, such as laparotomy, is a significant risk.

14. **1-e, 2-a, 3-d, 4-c, 5-b.** Although it is not clear if this is of any clinical significance, *Cryptococcus* is found at high levels in pigeon droppings, and there is a theoretical risk of contracting the disease from people with prolonged contact to pigeon droppings. Spelunking, or cave exploration, is a classic risk factor for *Histoplasma*, which is found at high concentrations in bat droppings. Administration of broad-spectrum antibiotics is a risk factor for invasive candidiasis. Metabolic acidosis, probably due to inhibition of host phagocytes, is the major risk factor for development of mucormycosis, an infection caused by *Mucor* or *Rhizopus*. Finally, *Sporothrix* is inoculated into the body after a skin break caused by thorns. The classic boards question is a gardener who develops fevers and ascending lymphadenopathy in one arm.

15. **b)** *Entamoeba* is the cause of amoebic liver abscess.

16. **1-b, 2-d, 3-a, 4-c.**

17. **d)** Tertian fevers occur on every 3rd day, or every 48 hr, while quartan fevers occur on every 4th day, or every 72 hr. The organisms which cause tertian fever, *P. vivax* and *P. ovale*, both reside in the liver. Chloroquine treats the blood-born merozoites, but does not penetrate into the dormant liver forms, allowing recrudescence to occur. Chloroquine plus primaquine should be used in such patients. Conversely, *P. malaria* causes quartan fevers and has no liver phase. It can be treated successfully with chloroquine alone. *P. falciprum* does cause the most severe malaria, due to higher organism burdon and the risk of microcapillary thrombosis in the

brain. Resistance to quinine derivatives is becoming a global problem.

18. **1-c, 2-d, 3-e, 4-b, 5-c, 6-a, 7-b.** *Diphyllobothrium* and *Clonorchis* are transmitted via ingestion of undercooked fish. *Echinococcus* can be transmitted from ingestion of eggs in dog feces or via consumption of undercooked sheep meat. Raw pork can transmit either *Taenia solium* or *Trichinella*, while raw beef can transmit *Taenia saginata* and raw crab meat can transmit *Paragonimus*.

19. **e)** Eosinophilia only occurs during infections caused by parasites that invade tissues. Tapeworms, for example, which only reside in the intestinal lumen, do not cause eosinophilia.

20. **1-i, 2-f, 3-h, 4-b, 5-a, 6-d, 7-e, 8-c, 9-g.**

21. **c)** The window period occurs when the immune system begins to clear viral antigens from the serum, but the antibody response has not yet achieved a titer which is detectable by lab assays. The immunodominant antigen of HBV is the surface antigen. Thus the window period is when the surface antigen has been cleared and thus is negative, but the titer of the surface antibody is not yet high enough to be detectable. Often during this period the antibody to the HBV core antigen is positive, as these antibodies seem to be produced earlier on. Thus the window period is typified by negative surface antigen, and positive core antibody, and negative surface antibody.

22. **1-h, 2-g, 3-i, 4-d, 5-a, 6-j, 7-e, 8-k, 9-b, 10-f, 11-c.**

INDEX

F

I

Q

R